Preconceptions: Preparation for
Pregnancy

PRECONCEPTIONS

Preparation for Pregnancy

PRECONCEPTIONS

Preparation for Pregnancy

Edited by
**John T. Queenan, M.D.,
and Kimberly K. Leslie, M.D.**

LITTLE, BROWN AND COMPANY

BOSTON   TORONTO   LONDON

Acknowledgments

I wish to thank the superb professional staff at Little, Brown and Company for their editing and publishing expertise. Special thanks go to Peggy L. Anderson for her editorial advice and devotion to this book. I wish to express my gratitude to Ray A. Roberts, who recognized the value of imparting this information to prospective parents. I greatly appreciate the secretarial help of Elizabeth M. Johnston, and, finally, I wish to thank Carrie Neher Queenan for her excellent editorial assistance.

FIRST EDITION

Library of Congress Cataloging-in-Publication Data

Preconceptions: preparation for pregnancy.
  Includes index.
    1. Pregnancy. I. Queenan, John T. II. Leslie,
Kimberly K.
RG525.P674 1989   618.2'4   89-12087

10 9 8 7 6 5 4 3 2 1

HC

Published simultaneously in Canada
by Little, Brown & Company (Canada) Limited

PRINTED IN THE UNITED STATES OF AMERICA

Contents

PRECONCEPTIONS

Preparation for Pregnancy

Introduction

THIS BOOK is about the beginning of life. So let me start at the beginning with the birth of a new approach to pregnancy.

In May 1985, Dr. Luella Klein gave her presidential address to the American College of Obstetricians and Gynecologists (ACOG) in Washington, D.C. What was momentous about this occasion? Dr. Klein was the first woman to be elected president of this professional organization. Having had a long history of working with teenage pregnancies, she felt very strongly that they were an unnecessary epidemic and therefore dedicated her tenure of office to decreasing the incidence of unwanted pregnancies. In order to develop this thrust, she invited Dr. David Grimes, then of the Centers for Disease Control in Atlanta, Georgia, to discuss the problem of "unwanted" pregnancies; and, because of our new preparation for pregnancy program at Georgetown University, she invited me to discuss the aspects of the "wanted" pregnancies.

In the United States, there are a total of 6 million pregnancies each year. Of these, approximately 900,000 abort spontaneously. An additional 1.5 million are terminated as induced abortions. This leaves approximately 3.6 million births each year in the United States. It would be totally naive to imagine that all of these births are wanted, much less planned. Trying to sort out whether a pregnancy is wanted or unwanted is very difficult. For the sake of discussion in our presentation, we divided pregnancies into three classifications: unwanted, mistimed, and intended. The unwanted pregnancies were those the couples clearly considered a mistake that resulted in a great deal of distress. The mistimed pregnancies were those in which couples were or were not using birth control and wished to have a child eventually, but had not planned a pregnancy at this moment. Finally, the intended pregnancies were those in which the couples wanted to have a baby, were not using any form of birth control, and anticipated the woman's becoming pregnant within the next few months.

I estimated that there were up to 2 million intended pregnancies each year in the United States, so being asked to participate in this ACOG program was a great challenge and opportunity. It was a challenge because we would be addressing three thousand practicing obstetricians and gynecologists from all over the United States. It was an opportunity because I knew there was a serious lack of resources for the couple who decided to become pregnant and wanted to make sure that all the conditions were optimal. Indeed, throughout our entire medical system, there were practically no organized provisions for this situation. Once a woman became pregnant, there were all sorts of pamphlets and courses — classes dealing with exercise during pregnancy, childbirth without anesthesia, taking care of the baby postpartum, and breast-feeding. But in fact, little or nothing existed for the couple who wanted to learn all of the factors that would give the best chance of a successful outcome to pregnancy *before* getting started. This forum would allow me to introduce our concept of the "twelve-month pregnancy," an approach to making sure systems are in the best order possible before conception.

So on that morning I stood before three thousand of my colleagues and issued a challenge. Nowhere in the United States, I pointed out, were there comprehensive resources for preparation for pregnancy. Yet, there were millions of couples each year who wished to have a comprehensive approach to information and evaluation. I outlined the program we had developed at Georgetown University, the first of its kind, which was started in 1984 to serve the many couples who wanted to begin a family and wanted to do everything possible to have an optimal outcome. The program, I told the audience, consisted of two evenings of short lecture presentations, with ample time for questions and answers. The course was directed by Dr. Kimberly Leslie and was taught by four obstetricians and gynecologists, a reproductive endocrinologist, a geneticist, a nurse, a financial administrator, and a nutritionist. They exercised great care to keep their remarks universal because some of the couples would be going to other doctors or delivering at other hospitals. The couples, I said, were also offered risk evaluation and physical examinations. The woman's blood was drawn for routine prenatal blood tests, which, I underscored, would ordinarily not be done until the first visit during pregnancy. Results of tests were available on the second evening so that they could be discussed with the couple.

I concluded my remarks by telling my colleagues that this was their opportunity to develop such programs in their offices or hospitals. These programs could be designed for their specific patient populations and would be an immense help in preparing couples for the most magnificent adventure they would ever undertake.

The response to this challenge has been very gratifying. Over the last four years, many hospitals, doctors' offices, and health associations have begun to offer preparation for pregnancy programs including education and risk evaluation. Some include physical examinations and laboratory evaluations. Numerous pharmaceutical companies have sponsored education programs. Although the response has not been universal, now there are many more resources available for couples wishing to prepare to have a baby.

We hope you will consider joining this partnership of couples and health professionals working together to make conditions optimal for pregnancy. To help you along, this book offers information similar to that provided in our prepregnancy program lectures. The two editors represent many years of specialized training and are qualified not only as obstetricians and gynecologists but also as specialists in maternal and fetal medicine. John T. Queenan brings the experience of two and one-half decades of practicing obstetrics. Kimberly K. Leslie brings the perspective of a woman two years after completion of a maternal-fetal medicine fellowship. Together, with the help of several colleagues, we will guide you through the new concept of preparation for pregnancy. Let us begin!

John T. Queenan, M.D.

[PART I]

Planning Your Pregnancy: Practical and Personal Considerations

[1]

The Case for Prepregnancy Planning

John T. Queenan, M.D.

Consider for a moment the awe and excitement created by President Kennedy's challenge to the United States to put a man on the moon in ten years. To accomplish this miraculous feat, so many factors had to be precise and so many events had to occur in perfect sequence. Nothing was more crucial than the preparation necessary for lift-off. Many intelligent people would have said it was impossible. But, as astronauts Armstrong and Aldrin might well remind us, that's all history now.

The gift of human reproduction is many times more complicated than putting a man on the moon. And yet more than 3.5 million babies are born each year in the United States alone. This represents almost ten thousand miracles a day. From conception to cell division to implantation to development of organ systems, a number of factors must occur with precision. It is logical to assume that what you do in preparation for conception will improve the chances of having a healthy baby. That is what this book is all about — the preparation for pregnancy.

INTELLIGENT PEOPLE like to approach new ventures with as much information as possible. Buy a new product and you receive a myriad of printed instructions to read prior to use. Fly in a commercial airplane and you will hear a litany of safety instructions that you could probably recite by heart. But how about having a baby? In the past, instructions, resources, and information in this area have been devoted largely to preparation for childbirth. Traditionally, information-gathering about a woman's pregnancy and the initial physician evaluation of her status have taken place well into the first trimester, or first three months of the pregnancy. In this book we present a new concept, preparation for pregnancy.

This chapter and those that follow will give you general background information covering all of the aspects of pregnancy and childbirth that a couple should be aware of before entering into the venture of having a baby. In addition, we will provide information for prospective parents concerning the importance of health histories, reproductive histories, physical examinations, screening procedures, and counseling. Each of these aspects is valuable in helping to prepare a couple for an optimal outcome to their pregnancy. This concept is new because the information, examination, and evaluation are provided prior to the onset of pregnancy. The next several pages will show you why prepregnancy planning can be vital to the well-being of your newborn child.

Consider this scenario. Ken and Joyce Brown are planning to have a baby and now Joyce's menstrual period is overdue. She calls the obstetrician's office and speaks to the receptionist. "Yes," Joyce is told, "it is possible that since your menstrual period is late you may be pregnant. You may want to give yourself a urinary pregnancy test to confirm this, but in any case Dr. Smith prefers to see patients after they miss their second menstrual period so that he is sure that the pregnancy is off to a good start." So Joyce obtains a urine pregnancy test kit from her local pharmacy, and indeed she has a positive test. She calls the doctor's office with this information and requests an appointment. The receptionist tells her that Dr. Smith is booked up at the time of her second missed menstrual period but they will work her into the schedule as soon thereafter as possible. Joyce is finally given an appointment for her initial physical examination for the tenth week after her last menstrual period.

Now, Joyce had planned to become pregnant and when, approximately two weeks after the beginning of her last menstrual period, she ovulated, one of the eggs was fertilized and she became pregnant. Within five days, the fertilized ovum had already divided several times and had implanted in her uterus. It is during the first eight weeks of pregnancy that organogenesis, or the formation of organs and organ systems, occurs and the fate of the fetal organs is determined. (It may be helpful to clarify here that *pregnancy* is calculated from the date of the last period; *conception* occurs about two weeks after the period. So organogenesis is complete six weeks after conception.) When Joyce arrived in the doctor's office, she was already ten weeks pregnant, and any information that would have been valuable in making conditions optimal for the growing embryo or that would have allowed her and Ken to avoid hazards was no longer useful.

Scheduling the initial prenatal examination after the second missed menstrual period is too late! By that time organogenesis is complete. Therefore, information on diet, medications, vitamins, hyperthermia, or exercise that might have prevented potential harm to the fetus is already worthless.

Why Prepregnancy Planning Is Vital:
Some Key Examples

Early in pregnancy, the embryo is exquisitely vulnerable to noxious stimuli like harmful drugs, viruses, environmental pollutants, or physical harm due to hyperthermia (overheating of the body) or radiation. As pregnancy progresses, stimuli that might have been noxious early in pregnancy may have little or no effect.

A scientific study possibly demonstrating the value of prepregnancy care in avoiding a specific problem that occurs during early pregnancy was recently conducted in Northern England, Scotland, Wales, and Ireland, where the incidence of neural tube defects (NTD, congenital defects involving the brain and spinal cord) is extremely high. The common NTDs include spina bifida (incomplete closure of the spinal column, exposing the spinal cord membranes and even the spinal cord) and anencephaly (incomplete development of the cerebrum and absence of the top of the fetal skull). The incidence of NTDs in that part of the world is as high as eight per thousand live births. In contrast, the incidence in the United States is one to two per thousand births. Once a family has one affected child, the recurrence rate is 3 percent to 5 percent (2 percent in the United States) with the next pregnancy. Should a couple have two infants in a row affected with a neural tube defect, the chances are as high as 10 percent in that part of the world that their next child will be affected also. The research emphasizing the importance of preparation prior to becoming pregnant was done by R. W. Smithells and investigators[1] and showed that the risk of recurrent NTDs could be decreased if multivitamins and folic acid (folate), a member of the B vitamin complex family, were taken

---

[1] Reported in *Lancet*, May 7, 1983.

twenty-eight days before a pregnancy and continued to the time of the second missed menstrual period. In Smithells's study, patients receiving full supplements of vitamins and folic acid were treated for at least twenty-eight days before the pregnancy. The vitamins and folic acid were discontinued at the time of the second missed menstrual period, or after organogenesis was complete. Another group of mothers received no vitamins or folate. Among the mothers who had one prior NTD and received full supplementation, the recurrence rate was 0.5 percent. Among the mothers who had one prior NTD and who received neither vitamins nor folate supplements, the recurrence rate was 4.2 percent. Among mothers having two children with NTDs and receiving full supplementation, the recurrence rate was 2.3 percent; unsupplemented mothers had a recurrence rate of 9.6 percent.

The overall recurrence rate of NTDs was found to be approximately five times higher for mothers who were not supplemented versus mothers who received vitamins and folate. Of the mothers who received vitamins and folate twenty-eight days prior to pregnancy and during the first eight weeks of pregnancy, 234 (0.9 percent) had NTDs in subsequent pregnancies. Among those who were not supplemented, 11 out of 215 (5.1 percent) had NTDs.

This study has received various criticisms, including its method of patient selection and the fact that NTDs have begun to decrease recently (probably because vitamin supplementation and improved nutrition have become normal patterns of life) in Britain. Nonetheless, the study of Smithells suggested that specific measures taken prior to becoming pregnant and early in pregnancy are key factors in the optimal outcome of pregnancy. It is this sort of information that makes us feel so strongly that prepregnancy preparation and care are vital. There are many other instances in which preparation prior to conception will ensure an optimal outcome. For example, if a mother has insulin-dependent diabetes mellitus, she has an increased risk of having a baby with congenital malformations such as congenital heart malformations or defects of the central nervous system. If the diabetes is poorly controlled and the mother has elevated blood sugars, the likelihood of a congenital malformation is increased. J. Pederson and co-investigators demonstrated that if the diabetes is well controlled before conception the incidence of congenital malformations can be reduced.[2] But a recent collaborative multicenter study of more than one thousand pregnant women has shown that despite close monitoring and good blood glucose control, diabetic women are at higher risk for having a child with birth defects than are nondiabetic women.[3] However, diabetic women who started monitoring blood glucose levels before or immediately after conception had far better outcomes than diabetic women who did not seek medical care until later in pregnancy.

The rubella virus (measles) is a well-known teratogen (an agent capable of producing congenital malformations). A mother contracting rubella during the first eight weeks of pregnancy stands an extremely high chance of having a baby with congenital malformations, which may involve deafness, blindness, and/or congenital heart disease, as well as many other problems. Today, 15 percent of women in their reproductive years are susceptible to rubella. Scientists know this because these women show no antibodies against rubella, the presence of which would indicate that they have been vaccinated against the disease or indeed have had rubella at some time in the past. A rubella-susceptible woman who becomes pregnant places her unborn child at considerable — and needless — risk. But if, prior to be-

[2] Reported in *British Medical Journal*, 1:18, 1979.
[3] Reported in *New England Journal of Medicine*, March 17, 1988.

coming pregnant, she were to be tested for rubella susceptibility, she would then have the opportunity to receive immunization if needed and eliminate the risk to her baby. Such a woman would have to avoid pregnancy for three months, because the virus may be shed from the cervix for that long after vaccination.

At one time, rubella-induced congenital malformations were relatively common. Fortunately, the energetic campaigns to immunize young people against rubella have markedly reduced the incidence of this problem today. It seems tragic that we can be aware of the possibility of preventing rubella, that we have all of the means at our disposal, yet there are still women who fail to achieve immunity prior to becoming pregnant, women who arrive pregnant in the doctor's office without having taken the precaution of finding out if they are immune to rubella. Ironically, these are often individuals who teach school or are in settings where they are exposed to many youngsters with rashes and illnesses that may raise the question of rubella.

Today, 2 to 3 percent of the population develop atypical blood group antibodies. These are antibodies that form in response to foreign red blood cell surface elements called antigens. In the case of a pregnant woman, this may occur from a spontaneous or induced abortion, a prior cesarean section, or, very infrequently, from a mismatched blood transfusion. If the fetus inherits the corresponding antigen on the red cells, the antibodies may destroy them, causing an anemia in the fetus. It is very important for a potential mother who has these irregular antibodies to know about this prior to conceiving. If she has Rh-negative blood and has anti-Rh antibodies (or if she is Kell negative and has anti-Kell antibodies), her chances of delivering future healthy babies are already compromised. This would be very valuable information for her, especially if a voluntary interruption of pregnancy were ever contemplated, because this current pregnancy might be her best chance to have a healthy baby. Subsequent pregnancies might pose even greater difficulties due to the buildup of blood group antibodies.

Finally, prepregnancy evaluation is crucial if there is any chance that either party is potentially infected with the AIDS virus. Because the mother affected by AIDS is likely to transmit the infection to her fetus, learning about such an infection may be a reason for her to decide not to become pregnant.

History and Physical Examination

The possibility of anticipating problems in a pregnancy is extremely good if a very careful evaluation of the couple's background is obtained prior to conception. Most obstetricians have a standard list of questions. For instance, a questionnaire covering the mother's past health and reproductive history could prove helpful. Are her menstrual cycles normal and regular? Does she have any major medical illnesses? Has she had prior surgery that might affect her ability to reproduce?

Likewise, information about the father is very important. Has he ever had any illnesses that would possibly leave him with a low sperm count? The classic example is mumps orchitis (inflammation of the testes). Additionally, are there any problems detected on physical examination that suggest there could be difficulty with fertility, for instance a varicocele (varicose veins in the scrotum)? What medications does he take or has he been exposed to in the past? Does he indulge in excessive alcohol? What about recreational drug use?

The physical exam of the potential mother is extremely valuable. If the complete physical examination reveals no abnormalities, one can anticipate she herself will do well when having her baby. It is common practice on the first office visit during pregnancy to do routine screening including a complete blood count, urinalysis, blood group, Rh, and tests for abnormal antibodies. Additional tests include a measurement of the rubella antibody level, a test for syphilis, a Pap smear, a gonorrhea culture, and hepatitis B surface antigen. Performing these tests is considered "routine" and good practice on the first prenatal visit.

Can we consider a better, more contemporary approach? If these tests were performed prior to pregnancy, many advantages would ensue. If the complete blood count reveals anemia, it is better treated prior to the onset of pregnancy. The developing fetus will do better with an adequate amount of maternal hemoglobin than having to cope with the mother's anemia. Likewise, a lump in the breast should obviously be evaluated and treated prior to pregnancy. A breast lump necessitating removal during pregnancy poses an increased risk of miscarriage, as does any surgery during the first trimester of pregnancy. If the urinalysis reveals a urinary tract infection, it is usually very easy to treat prior to pregnancy. The medications used to treat such infections are usually not a problem for a developing embryo, but why take the chance?

Serology is a test for syphilis. Today, this is a rare sexually transmitted disease. Nonetheless, it is a law in most states that a serologic test for syphilis be performed during pregnancy because of the devastating effects syphilis can have on the embryo and fetus. If all routine screening is done prior to pregnancy, this is the only test that needs to be repeated during pregnancy. Many states perform this free.

The Pap smear is capable of detecting early cellular changes in the cervix. Over a course of time, these cells may progress to preinvasive malignant-appearing cells and eventually even to cancer of the cervix. Since cancer of the cervix is a disease preventable by having Pap smears on a regular basis and by therapy for early abnormalities of the cervix, it is standard practice for women to undergo periodic Pap smears. If a woman for one reason or another put off having her regular Pap smear until after pregnancy began, finding it to be abnormal would be very unfortunate. Commonly the workup of an abnormal Pap smear requires evaluation by colposcopically directed biopsies, which are then examined under the microscope by the pathologist. If there is no malignancy, simple freezing of the cervix with a cryosurgery unit will be all that is needed to treat this problem. However, it is considerably more difficult to take biopsies of the cervix and perform cryosurgery on the pregnant uterus.

A polyp protruding from the cervical canal is another common problem. If this is detected prior to pregnancy, it is a very simple matter for the doctor to remove this polyp and submit it to the laboratory for pathologic evaluation. Again, it is more difficult to remove a polyp once a pregnancy has begun.

The detection of gonorrhea prior to conception affords the opportunity to treat this disease adequately without the risk to the embryo that can result from the administration of antibiotics during pregnancy. If the gonorrhea culture happens to be positive, follow-up tests are performed during pregnancy to prevent infection of the baby's eyes by the gonococcus bacteria at birth.

Genetic Screening

During pregnancy, it is common for your doctor to inquire about various predictable complications of reproduction that occur on a genetic basis (these are discussed in greater detail in Chapter 11). For instance, eastern European, Ashkenazi Jews may unknowingly be carriers for Tay-Sachs disease; that is, they have the abnormal gene but are not afflicted with the disease. If both parents are carriers, the chances are 1 in 4 that their child will be afflicted and will thus experience progressive mental and physical deterioration, until it dies, usually by age three. The presence of Tay-Sachs disease in the fetus can be detected with amniocentesis and amniotic fluid analysis. If the parents are tested prior to pregnancy, they can enter the pregnancy knowing if amniocentesis will be necessary. Because genetic amniocentesis is done fifteen to seventeen weeks into the pregnancy, having the Tay-Sachs carrier tests done before pregnancy can avoid a time crunch in the scheduling of this special procedure. (Amniocentesis is also described in Chapter 11.)

Hemoglobinopathies (abnormalities of the oxygen-carrying hemoglobin in red blood cells) occur in certain individuals. For instance, sickle cell hemoglobinopathies, which are responsible for a variety of ailments, occur predominantly in blacks; thalassemia hemoglobinopathies, which include severe, incurable anemia, occur in people of Mediterranean extraction (Greek, Italian). Testing for the carrier state or for the presence of these diseases is rather simple; it is preferably done before pregnancy so you will know if amniocentesis will be necessary.

Screening prior to pregnancy is important for individuals who have a family history of congenital malformations, unexplained stillborns, or mental retardation. In such cases, chromosome evaluations of the affected individuals may reveal chromosome abnormalities. Alternate forms of these abnormalities could exist in ostensibly normal individuals and be transmitted through reproduction in such a way that offspring are abnormal. (Incidentally, this situation is different from that in which mothers of advanced maternal age — thirty-five or older — may have chromosome abnormalities resulting from their age. These age-related problems can only be ruled out *during* pregnancy, by either chorionic villus sampling seven to nine weeks into the pregnancy or by genetic amniocentesis at fifteen to seventeen weeks.)

We have considered here what sounds to be an extensive amount of screening tests. But these are standard tests for all pregnancies. In the past, these have always been done on the first or subsequent prenatal visits. We propose that a couple wishing to start a pregnancy can improve chances for an optimal outcome by having this done *prior* to pregnancy. There is little or no increased cost, and the benefits can be enormous.

Prepregnancy Counseling

Prior to pregnancy, it is vital to have counseling in various areas that will help couples to achieve proper health habits and avoid certain harmful hazards. Many of these areas will be addressed in detail in later sections of this book. For instance, diet and exercise are very important considerations that are better addressed prior to becoming pregnant. Some people must take medications for an existing illness, and these should be reviewed very carefully prior to pregnancy. Some medications may have no ill effect, but others must be discontinued if they could be harmful. The consequences of smoking and using alcohol need to be considered, as well as exposure to certain environmental health hazards. The entire area of counseling is extremely important. If couples understand what constitutes risks and what constitutes improving the chance for having a healthy baby, they can make intelligent day-by-day decisions.

In addition, information regarding the signs and symptoms of pregnancy is important so that the couple knows what to expect. The mother should understand the symptoms of early pregnancy as well as some of the signs that occur as hormones cause mild to moderate changes in her breasts, body contours, and pelvic organs. The mother should be counseled concerning danger signs; for instance, spotting and cramping during early pregnancy may indicate a threatened miscarriage or an ectopic pregnancy. Because modern pregnancy tests and diagnostic ultrasound enable the obstetrician to differentiate these rather early, the evaluation of these clinical situations is markedly improved today. Nonetheless, a mother who does not know what to expect is at a distinct disadvantage in knowing when to contact her doctor.

Understanding the physiology of pregnancy for both prospective parents is important. Since some of the symptoms of early pregnancy may be rather troublesome or occasionally even incapacitating, the couple should be aware of what to expect. On balance, pregnancy is a normal physiologic event, and most mothers go through it with few or no problems. But, adequate knowledge in this area is extremely important to an enjoyable and healthy pregnancy.

Treatment

In general, if the mother's health history and prepregnancy physical examination reveal no areas of special concern, such as those outlined above, medical treatment prior to pregnancy is seldom necessary. The one exception is that we strongly recommend standard prenatal vitamins containing iron and folic acid. The work of Smithells and co-investigators is impressive. While it is very difficult to prove that we are increasing the chance of an optimal pregnancy outcome, reflecting on that study gives us some reassurance that prenatal vitamins containing folic acid are at least very helpful. These should be started before the onset of pregnancy to assure adequate levels. Occasionally, nausea and vomiting in the first trimester make taking vitamins difficult. A woman's need for extra iron during pregnancy is well established. Other therapy should be included, as appropriate, if an abnormality is detected in the prenatal evaluation. Otherwise, no other specific therapy is indicated.

With good information and the program that is presented in this book, a couple can collaborate in a magnificent experience, that of having a child. They can be assured that they are doing everything possible to ensure that the outcome of the pregnancy is a healthy mother and a healthy baby.

[2]

Your Personal Situation: Job, Home, Family
Carrie Neher Queenan, B.A.

Having a baby is a magnificent undertaking. No other experience will cause such profound changes in your life. Your relationship to your spouse, friends, fellow workers, and (most important) to an older child will take on new dimensions. Happily, most of the changes brought about by having a baby will be positive and will make your relationships with other people even more meaningful. And, of course, your child will return your love and affection many times over.

Let us not imply that having a baby does not entail increased responsibilities and even some difficulties and heartaches — all of this comes along with the joys. Having a child requires the acceptance of many new obligations. Soon you come to the realization that you have created someone who is totally dependent upon you for many years.

Your life will change in many ways, and it is important to understand as much as you can about this so that you can plan ahead. Planning will give you peace of mind and help to eliminate many of the mysteries and fears that come with the unknown. In addition, learning what lies ahead will help you to organize the support systems that are absolutely essential if you are to adapt successfully to your challenging new life-style. As you will

*see in this chapter on personal considerations, assessing your
need for support systems and organizing them ahead of time will
be very valuable to you.*

T HE REALIZATION that you are planning to bring
a new person into the world is bound to produce a mixture
of feelings and a variety of new life situations. There is no
one set of rules, no one set of answers that applies to
everyone, for this is a very individual time. Being pregnant
is a state of health that is natural and normal. It should
be a time of excitement, well-being, and joy. This is, however, a period of major changes necessitating the development of a life-style that accommodates the needs of the
developing baby and the emotional and physical needs of
the prospective parents. This chapter will address some of
the aspects of your personal situation that you will need
to consider when planning to have a baby.

Reactions to pregnancy may vary widely from person to
person, *and* from moment to moment in the same individual. The woman who learns she is pregnant may be happy
about the prospect of having a baby one day, unhappy the
next day, and uncertain about the whole thing the next;
the prospective father may find his feelings shifting from
pride to anxiety to ambivalence. All of this is normal and
to be expected. How you react to pregnancy will be influ-
enced by your age, previous life experience, social background, and your emotional and physical comfort level
with yourself, others, and your physician. Today, women
are more curious and more knowledgeable than ever about
their health. They want to know what is happening.

For the couple who are becoming parents for the first
time, there is so much to learn, and so many changes lie
ahead. Today, approximately 65 percent of women between the ages of twenty-two and forty-eight work outside

the home. Nearly half of all children under the age of six have a mother who works. It is more than likely your pregnancy will be planned. It is also likely you will become involved in a very challenging juggling act between your job demands, your emotional and physical needs, your partner's feelings, and the impact of changing financial and space requirements as a result of your decision to have a baby.

At home, both partners may experience mood swings. Normal hormonal changes and fatigue are obvious causes for the woman's experience. The father worries about his ability to provide for mother and child. Understanding that these changes are not unusual for either partner and that your disposition will return to normal certainly will help you cope with the immediate peaks and valleys. Sharing your feelings and needs and reassuring one another is not only comforting, it contributes to the development of a strong family unit. Actually, this time may represent a significant period of maturation for your relationship as a couple.

Job Considerations

In the workplace, accommodations become necessary. When you are pregnant, there may be schedule changes as you need to alter your pace, to get off your feet, travel less, and work shorter hours. Don't forget, you will make ten to fifteen visits to the obstetrician's office! All this has an impact upon your employer and your co-workers, whose acceptance and cooperation you desire. The extent of your interactions and interdependence with your co-workers will determine, to a great degree, their reaction to your news. No matter how well you plan to cover your job responsibilities, your colleagues will perceive that they will have to share your load. Therefore, considerable thought should be given to how and when to tell your co-workers about your pregnancy. The appropriate time for breaking the news could be after the first trimester, when chances of miscarriage have markedly decreased.

In 1978, Congress passed the Pregnancy Discrimination Act, which ruled that pregnancy must be treated in the same manner as any other medical condition. Therefore, an individual who becomes pregnant cannot be singled out or discriminated against for resulting absence or disability. For example, if employee A contracts hepatitis and as part of the treatment is ordered by his physician to stay at bed rest for three months, and employee B is found to have placenta previa (a placenta abnormally implanted over the cervix) and is similarly confined to bed for three months, the employer is required to treat both situations equally.

The handling of disability varies among employers; check with your personnel (or human resources) department. If your employer offers no compensation, you may qualify for temporary benefits from your state. The local unemployment office is the best place for you to find out about the specific benefits available in your area.

The question of maternity leave will arise. Although currently three of four women are likely to experience pregnancy during their working lives, no national policy regarding guaranteed maternity leave exists in the United States. Maternity benefits are left to the employer's discretion. Since women compose the majority of the work force, chances are good your company will have a maternity leave policy. Learn the details of your company's policies before you enter into negotiations. Six to eight weeks off after the birth of a baby is becoming customary. Often additional time off without pay can be secured. Similar leave options should be available to adoptive parents.

At this time, there is no universal practice in the United States regarding paternity leave. Basically, this is an issue of economics for the employer, so the larger the company or corporation, the more likely the opportunity for some type of leave. Taking leave without pay or using vacation days are ways a father can arrange time at home. The amount of time a father chooses or is able to stay at home will vary according to many outside factors. What really matters is the quality of time spent with his new family, not the amount of days taken off from work. Obviously, there are emotional and psychological benefits as well as practical advantages for all if the father is free to be part of the home scene. Practically speaking, there will be errands to run, family and friends to greet, chores to be done; performing such tasks will increase the father's sense of involvement and give the mother a chance to rest. Cuddling, changing, and feeding the baby can be joyous experiences promoting further bonding between father and child. Sharing in the care of the baby and the joys of this time will do much to prevent or at least decrease any sense of isolation a father may have when surrounded by the all-encompassing female experience of motherhood.

Plan leave time with your specific situation in mind. If you will be taking six weeks of maternity leave, it may be preferable for you to be off two weeks prior to your delivery date, leaving almost four weeks at home after the baby has arrived. Nowadays, shorter hospital stays — usually two days (down from five days) for a regular delivery, and three days (down from seven days) for a cesarean section — afford greater time at home. Obviously, the best way to allocate such time will vary with each household. Is this your first child or are there other children needing you? Will you have help — for a few days, weeks, part-time, full-time, live-in? Will other family members share in child care responsibilities? Have you planned any time just for yourself?

Is working until the end of pregnancy a realistic expectation? Many factors will influence this decision. Your own preference and financial needs immediately come to mind. The status of your overall health, the progress of your pregnancy, your age, and your life-style must be considered. The type of work you do, number of hours involved, factors leading to stress and fatigue, job related and environmental threats to your fetus — all of these are issues to review. Do not, however, lose sight of the fact that pregnancy is, for most women, a healthy condition.

A pregnancy may give rise to concern about the future of your career and that of your partner. If this is a planned pregnancy and you have control, develop an overall life plan. Review your personal priorities. Discuss and determine your goals and priorities as a couple. Timing is often a key factor. Once your reputation has been established, it becomes less necessary to prove yourself to your employer and colleagues. Delaying parenthood may allow time to carve out a professional identity. Achieving senior status or advanced skills could allow taking extended time away — even several years — to have children. A woman with seniority is likely to have an easier time reentering the professional arena.

What to Expect During Pregnancy: An Overview

Today, when fewer people are surprised by becoming pregnant, it is logical to conclude that a couple has spent some emotional energy discussing feelings about work and parenthood. It is well to remember that everyone brings his or her own set of family experiences and perceptions to the consideration of these roles. Openness and sensitivity will be good allies when exchanging thoughts about the appropriateness of each partner's role as a parent and as a productive individual.

During the first trimester, feelings of excitement are commonly mingled with bouts of ambivalence. You have made a momentous decision. Telling each other of your feelings can help lessen the anxieties that are often associated with your self-perception, your ability to cope, and your capacity to handle *all* of the new demands. It is a time to promote a dialogue with your partner that will enable you both to gain perspective during this period of many changes. Enrolling in childbirth classes provides an excellent opportunity for both partners to learn and practice skills needed during labor and birth, to share information and experiences with others in similar circumstances, and to become familiar with what will happen during your actual delivery and hospitalization.

As an expectant mother, you may be plagued by nausea at work or during meal preparation. The need to urinate frequently is a bother, often interrupting precious sleep — sleep that is hard to catch up on during the day and increasingly difficult at night as breast tenderness prevents resting in your favorite position. Management of your appearance takes ingenuity as your regular clothing becomes uncomfortable. This could get increasingly complicated for you, since you may not yet have disclosed that you are pregnant!

The second trimester usually offers some relief. Nausea is disappearing or totally gone. Your body seems to have adjusted to the hormonal changes, and there is a general feeling of calm and well-being. Travel becomes much easier, with few if any restrictions likely to be imposed. You can feel the baby move and you will begin to look pregnant. There is praise, acceptance, and support for your pregnancy from those around you. You are likely to get a reprieve from fatigue. Be alert, however, to the possibility of growing anxiety on the part of the father as the development of the baby becomes increasingly apparent. Reassure him. Share with each other. If a genetic amniocentesis or sonogram is to be done, it will most likely take place during this trimester. The sonogram allows you to view your baby in the uterus, presenting a special opportunity for early parental bonding.

Throughout the third trimester, your baby will continue to grow and gain weight. You will feel "big" and your activities are likely to become more limited. Some travel restrictions may be imposed as your due date draws near. Additional rest periods will be welcome. Slight swelling of your feet is bothersome but normal. Propping them up for periods during the day, or lying down, will help to make you more comfortable.

It is now time to start preparing yourself and your home for the baby's arrival. Select and pack the basic necessities for the hospital. Make sure you tell your partner and family where they are! Preparation of living space for the baby is thrilling, but also hard work. Share this special endeavor with the father.

Both parents will experience bouts of excitement and anxiety as the time approaches. Exasperation may best describe your state if your pregnancy continues beyond your due date. Do not forget that the more you know about your type of delivery and your hospital's procedures and facilities (more on this is in Chapter 3), the greater your comfort level at the time of the baby's birth.

Remember, health is a family affair. Ideally, having both parents striving to be physically and emotionally fit, rested, and free of any toxins such as alcohol, drugs, and cigarettes provides the best start for a baby. Familiarizing yourself with the information in Part III of this book would be a big step in the right direction. The expectant mother should maintain a well-balanced diet, avoiding fatty foods, too many sweets, and convenience foods that provide poor nutrition. This often becomes harder as your pregnancy progresses and your life becomes increasingly hectic. Being physically strong before you conceive should provide a good foundation for a comfortable and active pregnancy.

If You Already Have a Child

Even if you already have a child and are planning a second baby, preparation is still the key. The mother's body's needs and reactions are likely to be similar to the first pregnancy; so the father and mother, as a result of their previous experience, are better able to recognize and comprehend the normal symptoms of pregnancy. However, some parents are troubled by the fact that each pregnancy, indeed, may be different. In this situation, seeking reassurance from your physician or appropriate family and friends will help you believe that you are capable of making the needed adjustments and accommodations. The excitement mingled with ambivalence, discussed earlier, is still possible. Becoming parents for a second time obviously increases the complexity of life management.

Along with the joyous anticipation comes the reality of increased financial responsibilities. The economic plans made when your first child was expected may now seem inadequate. A second child may involve greater costs for household help as well as expansion or rearrangement of your home to provide additional space. All of this may be added to existing obligations associated with schooling for your older child. It is normal to be anxious about these mounting challenges; it is normal to have arguments over your concerns. It is healthy to develop solutions together.

There are also additional emotional considerations. You may wonder if you really have enough love in your heart to share equally with another child. The father, while being proud, may also be increasingly jealous, since this time he knows what a personal and all-consuming experience motherhood is. He may remember the sensation of being on the sidelines, of feeling helpless and isolated during the early months of the first baby's entry into the family. This may be especially true if the mother breast-fed the baby.

He may have great anxiety related to the fear of losing his wife in childbirth, particularly when there is another child to care for. Sensitivity to these feelings and the current trends to involve the father throughout the pregnancy, labor, and rearing of the child are invaluable in helping him to feel included and to deal with his doubts and worries.

You also need to consider the effects of a new pregnancy on your first child. Real confusion and concerns can develop in the mind of even the very young. What is happening to Mommy? Is she sick? Will she leave me? It is crucial to be aware of the dynamics of this changing relationship. Let the child share in the wonder of the growth of the baby. Include your child in the visits to the doctor's office. Let him listen to the baby's heartbeat. Show him the hospital where Mommy will go. Share your plans; tell him who will care for him, where he will be and for how long when Mommy is in the hospital. Involve the father in these exchanges, which are designed to provide loving and frequent reassurances. Little gifts for the child at home can ease the pain of separation and serve as reminders of Mommy's continuing love while she is in the hospital.

A certain amount of regression is normal and to be expected as attention to the new baby intrudes on your other child's world. Toilet training often experiences a setback. Behavior may become more juvenile and sleep patterns may change. Be aware of the jealousy that can develop long before the baby is born and is certain to be a part of the picture when the baby comes home. Talking about what is happening will soothe these concerns and is key to their resolution. A visit to the hospital to see Mommy and meet the new baby may be very comforting for all.

Overcoming Pregnancy Loss

Planning a pregnancy after having experienced pregnancy loss, or after your baby has died, needs some discussion. This loss has tremendous impact. The situation may be more readily dealt with, at least by others, if an infant was involved than if the loss was a miscarriage. To the parents, however, such a loss — whenever it occurs — often evokes anger at oneself, each other, and the outside world. Time is an important factor in the healthy resolution of such grief. Sharing your feelings with those who understand (for example, support groups, others who have suffered similar loss, or special counselors) will lessen the pain and bring some comfort. Many hospitals have bereavement counselors and special programs. There is a wealth of literature dealing with loss, directed to mothers, fathers, children of all ages, extended families, and care givers.

Being ready for another pregnancy depends on many factors: your state of health, the emotional recovery of you and your partner, and the quality and stability of your relationship, to cite a few. When you are ready to become pregnant again, the fear and anxiety resulting from your previous loss will be greatly reduced if you become as knowledgeable as possible about your chances for a successful pregnancy. Although many couples never feel totally safe until a subsequent pregnancy has been completed, your confidence should be increased by knowing that when you lose a baby due to a nonrecurring cause, you have an overwhelming chance of a favorable outcome for your next pregnancy. By sorting out your old feelings, you will gain new perspectives leading to a renewed feeling of well-being.

What if You Have Problems Conceiving?

For the couple experiencing problems with infertility, planning a pregnancy can be an emotional roller coaster. There is the desire to get all in order and ready, but you hesitate to proceed, as your constant hope has been thwarted by frequent failures. Infertile couples often develop a sense of helplessness and loss of control. Much emotional energy is invested in the goal of childbearing. According to Melvin L. Taymor, M.D., when that goal is frustrated by delays or losses and the couple begins to sense that they may be unable to bear a child, an emotional state labeled the crisis of infertility often develops. This state affects all areas of their life together — social, psychological, moral, and religious. The crisis can manifest itself in various forms of anxiety, frustration, depression, guilt, obsession, and isolation. The couple's emotional turmoil can affect the biological process so that a vicious circle of failure to conceive is established. Physicians should recognize and treat the *total* problem of infertility.

Tremendous advances have been made in the treatment of infertility, and many ways to successful childbearing are available. A discussion of the technical aspects is not appropriate here (see chapter 5). However, there are some personal considerations. Seeking treatment from a qualified specialist is most important. In addition, couples undergoing the basic workup for infertility should be open to the option of meeting with an infertility counselor, who should be trained in dealing with psychological aspects of infertility. This interviewer may be in a better position than the physician to elicit detailed and often guarded information. In front of the doctor, a couple may prefer to present a good picture and may withhold information and deny feelings. Attending a series of orientation conferences in which the facts of reproduction, infertility tests, and treatment are presented to several couples at once can relieve anxiety, clarify misinformation, and reduce the patients' feeling of helplessness. The options for support are many — individual sessions, group counseling, visits with the woman alone or with her partner, whatever best suits your set of circumstances.

Thinking of the positive things you can do and engaging in constructive activities are effective elixirs. Even though you are obviously less certain when you will become pregnant, get your body ready. A good diet and an appropriate fitness regime are positive activities. It is very beneficial to share your anxieties with your partner and others with similar problems. You will be overjoyed at the news of your conception, but do not be surprised if you then experience feelings of ambivalence. Mixed feelings are normal.

Obviously, many different life scenarios are possible. We hope this discussion has answered some questions, presented some useful suggestions, and started you thinking about your very individual and personal situation. There is help. Useful programs and information for just about any imaginable combination of needs are readily available. It is up to you to go after them. By reading this book, you have already started.

Planning a pregnancy, regardless of numerous varieties of personal circumstance, involves challenges and change. Organization, cooperation, communication, and sufficient support systems are the essential elements of successful management for a couple with the demands of careers and children. There is often a fine line between an exciting, vigorous, full life and a horrible rat race. Love, support, flexibility, preparation, and planning are the keys to keeping sane. Allow yourself time to reflect, get some perspective, and then expend the energy to make the necessary changes. Realize there are some things you can control and some you simply cannot. Concentrate on what you can control. What you are planning is the most special gift of life.

[3]

Choices
C. Lynne Queenan, B.A.

In the past, rules for pregnant mothers were strict and hospital regulations were almost inhumane. In the 1950s and 1960s, the scene started to change. The first important innovation was Grantly Dick-Read's advocacy of natural childbirth. Then, the Lamaze psychoprophylaxis for labor and delivery became popular. Fathers began to support their wives in labor, and finally they became part of the team in the delivery room. Today, most hospitals have abandoned their strict policies and have developed flexible attitudes toward the birth process. Your doctor and hospital will present you with many choices in having a baby. These are only some of the choices you will be facing, for as a couple you will be involved in many decisions from the time you begin planning to have a baby. Lynne Queenan discusses a range of important choices in this chapter.

HAVING A BABY is an exciting and profound opportunity. There are many decisions you will face that can make the experience a personal creative adventure, an experience that results in the most precious of all things — a new life.

Almost 90 percent of American women having babies have healthy, normal pregnancies. This chapter is for this often overlooked majority who share a commonality of experience and concerns. Studies show that three key issues bind this group together: 1) the desire for knowledge and understanding of the physiological and psychological changes experienced throughout pregnancy and childbirth, 2) the need for respect of their individual wishes concerning participation and approach to delivery, and 3) a concern for health maintenance as well as screening for early detection of any complications. The special aspects of high-risk situations will be covered in later chapters. However, the universality of the information presented here will, to a great degree, apply to most women preparing for pregnancy.

A review of some of the choices surrounding childbirth will give you an overview of what lies ahead. Hopefully, this will provide some insight into the decisions you can make to create an experience that is as meaningful and successful as possible.

Sharing the Experience

In the past, the father's role in preparation for pregnancy was very limited. After conception, his next major responsibility was getting the mother to the hospital when she went into labor. Today's environment and expectations are totally different, and fathers as well as mothers are now preparing for pregnancy. Often, a couple having a baby starts working as a team while planning for pregnancy and continues this tandem effort throughout the pregnancy, labor, delivery, and childrearing. The father's love, comfort, and support throughout the pregnancy and childbirth can greatly reduce the mother's stress, which, studies have shown, has a profound effect on the delivery and outcome.

When to Get Pregnant

Certainly, the timing of pregnancy is very important. The majority of American women work outside the home, and career decisions often affect the time they choose to start a family. Most significant is the fact that your child is wanted; and that you and your partner are doing everything within your power to make things perfect.

While it is important to give major attention to career needs, it is equally important to remember that age has ramifications on conception. The question of age, on balance, is outweighed by factors such as life-style, general health, fitness, and well-being of the partners. It is important for both partners to encourage health promotion and disease prevention during the preconception period. A woman in optimal condition begins her pregnancy with no drug use — no prescription or nonprescription medications, no social or illegal drugs, no tobacco or alcohol. She should also be exercising regularly, eating properly, and planning for continual prenatal care.

A couple must carefully consider all the factors related to pregnancy. For example, as later chapters will point out, infertility and chromosome anomalies tend to increase with age. Yet, the statistics are not as grim as you may believe. A woman giving birth at age forty still has a less than 1 percent chance of giving birth to a baby with Down syndrome. At the Centers for Disease Control, Dr. David Grimes conducted a study reviewing the birth records of more than twenty-six thousand women of all ages. He concluded that a higher rate of infant mortality did not exist for older women giving birth.

Couples today can often predict when ovulation is occurring by following cervical mucus changes or by using a simple urine test bought at a pharmacy. Ovulation prediction, detailed in Chapter 5, has important implications for optimal pregnancy outcome. By pinpointing ovulation, you can choose to get pregnant when conditions are ideal. For instance, if you were planning a pregnancy and developed a viral illness, such as an upper respiratory infection or influenza, you could then wait until the next cycle to conceive, thus avoiding any problem the virus might cause.

Choosing the Hospital

Even before pregnancy begins, it is wise to start researching hospital options. If there are no significant risk factors affecting the pregnancy, the choice of hospital usually makes little difference from a strictly medical standpoint. You have the opportunity to choose a hospital with facilities that fulfill your expectations. What used to be thought of as alternative birthing centers (such as birthing rooms, comfortable non–operating room surroundings) are options now offered by many hospitals in an effort to establish a more family-oriented environment. Whether you choose a small community hospital or a large general hospital probably will not make a difference in terms of safety for you or your baby, as long as the hospital is reputable. The Department of Health and Human Services now publishes the safety records of U.S. hospitals and makes this information available to the public through the Government Printing Office and local libraries.

If, however, there are factors making yours a high-risk pregnancy, the choice of a hospital becomes critical. You need to have a hospital with the ability to treat a complicated pregnancy as well as provide intensive maternal and newborn care. Such a hospital usually has in-hospital, around-the-clock anesthesia coverage, a laboratory and blood bank staffed twenty-four hours a day, maternal-fetal medicine physicians, and a newborn intensive care unit. It is important to note differences in hospital personnel and their availability, not just the equipment the institutions offer.

The reason for choosing the hospital before the physician is simple. If your pregnancy is high risk, you may limit your options by selecting a doctor who does not have admitting privileges at an appropriate hospital. Participating in a preparation for pregnancy program will facilitate the choice of a hospital and a doctor because risk evaluation is part of the program.

Choosing Your Health Care Provider

The most crucial decision you make may be determining who will deliver your baby. If you have a high-risk pregnancy, you may choose or be referred by your health care provider to a physician with special training; if your pregnancy is a normal one, you have a number of other options. Many different types of health care workers deliver babies. It is important to be aware of the level of training of your health care provider, since not all are trained to manage complicated, high-risk pregnancies. A family practitioner, for example, generally requires three years of training after medical school to be eligible for American Board of Family Practice certification. Approximately five months of that training is devoted to obstetrics and gynecology.

An obstetrician-gynecologist is required to take four years of residency training following medical school in order to be eligible to take the written exam for certification by the American Board of Obstetrics and Gynecology. Obstetricians passing the written exam are then eligible to apply for an oral exam, following one year of unsupervised practice. If they pass the oral exam, including a review of one year of their practice, they are then certified. Beginning in 1986, ten-year "time limited" certification was initiated. Board-certified obstetricians and gynecologists now need to undergo recertification every ten years.

Maternal-fetal medicine physicians are board-certified obstetrician-gynecologists who take two more years of specialty training in high-risk pregnancies. Afterward, they must take a written exam. If they pass, they must then take an oral exam after one year of unsupervised practice in this subspeciality. If they pass both exams, they are board-certified maternal-fetal medicine specialists.

The discussion above outlines three levels of training and proficiency. The family practitioner is not trained to manage the complicated high-risk pregnancy, while the maternal-fetal medicine specialist is trained to manage the most complicated cases. Meanwhile, the obstetrician-gynecologist is trained to manage normal and more complicated pregnancies.

Another option is to be delivered by a nurse-midwife. Nurse-midwifery generally requires one to two years of training in addition to nursing training. Basic nurse's training can last as few as three years or as many as five or six years, depending upon whether the nurse went to a diploma school or a degree school. Nurses who study midwifery are certified by the American College of Nurse Midwives. They are trained to take care of normal pregnancies. Certified nurse-midwives perform in a variety of settings, from home to hospital. Most commonly, they work in association with doctors. Knowing which doctor is associated with the midwife is vital, since complicated pregnancies will be referred to the physician.

The choice of one physician over another is a very personal matter. Obviously, you will want someone who is sensitive and instills confidence. You will also want a skilled professional whose manner and temperament are compatible with yours.

Various ways of selecting a physician are effective. If you have an internist or another physician whom you trust, he or she may be helpful in recommending an obstetrician with good credentials who would be compatible with your personality. Or, your friends may have had excellent experience with their doctors. These sorts of recommendations are invaluable. Finally, you can use the *Directory of Medical Specialists,* published for the American Board of Medical Specialists by Marquis Who's Who and available in most libraries. This lists biographies of all certified medical specialists, including their age, medical school, amount of training, professional societies, and hospital affiliations. But if you are looking up physicians who are just out of training, they will not be in the directory, since specialists cannot take their oral board examinations until after they have been in practice for over one year.

A word of caution is in order here regarding directories of doctors. Recently, doctor telephone referral services have sprung up in many cities. This is not the ideal way to choose an obstetrician, since many of these services operate on a fee-for-referral basis (for example, fifty dollars paid by the doctor for each new patient). Others are run by specific hospitals and recommend only physicians with admitting privileges at their hospitals.

Scheduling Your Health Care

If you work, the scheduling of your doctor's appointments can be critical. For instance, it may be impossible to leave your job in the middle of the day for a doctor's appointment. By arranging to be the first patient in the morning session, you may be able to see the doctor before you go to work. Similarly, if you schedule your visit for the last appointment of the day, you could miss as little time at work as possible. Some doctors now offer flexible evening office hours once or twice a week and others are open on Saturday. This is important to consider, since you may be making up to fifteen trips to the doctor during your pregnancy. While employers are usually understanding initially, frequent absences will not ingratiate you with your boss or peers.

Still, whatever you decide, it will take some juggling of your work schedule to fit in the dozen or so prenatal visits. If you have a time crunch, tell the nurse or scheduling secretary. This person can be a life (and job) saver. For instance, if the doctor is out delivering a baby in the middle of office hours (those are the realities), someone can call you before you leave work so that you won't have to waste your valuable time sitting in the waiting room.

A couple of tips are important here. In budgeting your time, you should be aware that the initial visit to the doctor's office includes a complete health history, physical exam, and laboratory tests. All of these take time. Subsequent visits are brief, focusing on blood pressure, weight, growth of the fetus, and urine checks for sugar or protein. You can get in and out of the office quickly if you don't spend a lot of time in the waiting room. Remember to bring along a list of any questions you may have so you can get them answered then and there.

A word about phone calls to your doctor. If you have reason to call during office hours or over the weekend, chances are your doctor will not be immediately available, unless it is an emergency. Do not wait to call until just before you have to go somewhere away from the telephone. Call early enough that you allow the physician time to call you back. Tell the nurse or answering service that you need to speak to the doctor and that you will be available at a certain phone number at specific times.

Labor Routines

As the time for your delivery approaches, your doctor will instruct you about the signs of labor and when in the process you should call him or her, depending upon your medical circumstances and the time it takes you to reach the hospital. For most women, labor begins with regular uterine contractions spaced far apart, perhaps every fifteen minutes. Over the next few hours, the contractions progress in frequency, duration, and intensity. There may be some bloody mucus (bloody show). Generally, mothers are told to go to the hospital when the frequency of contractions is under every ten minutes. The doctor will notify the hospital to expect your arrival. First labors average about thirteen hours in duration; subsequent labors are usually shorter.

In medicine, certain routines are followed to assure orderly procedures and good outcomes, the way a pilot goes through an equipment safety checklist before takeoff. But there are also some routines that may not be necessary or beneficial. These gray areas allow room for choices to be made with your partner and/or doctor. Such is the case with hospital labor routines.

Some physicians have standard admission orders. For instance, the physician may routinely order a shaving prep of the pubic hair and an enema on admission to the delivery floor. Shaving the pubic hair has no bearing on the outcome of the delivery; it is unnecessary. If your colon is not full, an enema is also not necessary. An intravenous infusion (IV) is another routine followed by some doctors. One advantage to the placement of an IV infusion during labor is to allow safe and quick intravenous access in case of an emergency. The IV also provides necessary hydration for the longer labor course. If you are a low-risk patient with the expectation of a reasonably short labor, it may not serve any purpose. These are areas that you may wish to discuss with your doctor before you go into labor so you may make your preferences known.

Pain Management During Labor

Participation in childbirth education classes does not decrease the duration of labor or reduce the risk of complications; it does, however, have a tremendously positive psychological effect. A 1986 study by M. E. Broome and C. Koehler, published in the journal *Family Community Health*, showed that women who participated in childbirth education programs used less pain medication, felt less pain, and reported more positive birth experiences than women who did not undergo similar training. Prepared fathers experienced a deep sense of involvement and attachment resulting from their training. The couple feels empowered by their motivated participation in the birth process.

There are many options for coping with pain during labor. Psychoprophylaxis is the suppression of physical pain associated with natural childbirth. Several methods to cope with pain exist, such as using hypnosis, soothing music, and visualization. One approach, pioneered by Dr. Grantly Dick-Read, is based on the theory that fear and tension produce pain. Dick-Read's method of childbirth preparation involves three aspects: educating the mother about the anatomy and physiology of childbirth, teaching her relaxation and breathing exercises, and, foremost to his theory, developing a "therapeutic relationship" between the woman and her doctor.

Perhaps the most popular method of pain management is Lamaze training, which enables the woman to relax and cope with the increasing strength of contractions. Relaxation techniques benefit the mother mentally and physically. Fear and anxiety are reduced and coping mechanisms are enhanced. The positive effects of relaxation include slowing down the breathing and heart rate, lowering the blood pressure, and maximizing the blood flow to the uterus, placenta, and fetus.

Lamaze classes involve both partners, usually starting around the seventh month of pregnancy with weekly two-hour sessions. Both partners receive instruction in breathing methods and relaxation techniques. You learn what to expect in labor and delivery, and your partner is taught comforting, supportive measures to lessen the pain of your labor. For many women, this is all that is necessary. For others, this works up to a certain point. If the contractions become too painful, pain medication will sometimes restore a woman's ability to concentrate and relax so she can continue with Lamaze techniques. Remember, no two labors are the same.

The differences between labors reside in the four P's: passage (size and shape of the pelvis), passenger (size of the baby), powers (strength of contractions), and psyche (the mother's mental attitude toward labor). If Lamaze has been used successfully but labor is long and hard, pain medicine will be a valuable help in coping with the labor. Pain medicine is generally safe when it is given at the proper time during labor. However, there is a definite limit to the amount of medicine that can be administered, because it crosses the placenta and enters fetal circulation.

Epidural anesthesia is a form of pain relief that has become popular with both patients and physicians. A slender needle is inserted into your back, between the vertebrae, at the level of your beltline. The needle does not enter the spinal canal, but stops short of it in what is called the epidural space. A test dose of anesthetic is instilled. If it is tolerated, the anesthesiologist then inserts a fine polyethylene catheter into the back so that anesthetic solution can be injected periodically. The epidural anesthetic takes away all or most of the pain. The results are usually dramatic. For those with hard labors, this is a superb means of relief for both labor and delivery. However, there are some drawbacks. Epidural anesthesia can decrease the strength of contractions, so that oxytocin (a hormone that induces uterine contractions) stimulation of labor may be necessary. It also takes away the sensation of the need to bear down and push the baby out during the second stage of labor, so the anesthesia may need to wear off before effective pushing can begin.

A lesser form of anesthetic relief, the pudendal block, is also effective. It is usually administered on the delivery table when you are ready to deliver. By anesthetizing the pudendal (external genital) nerves, there is substantially less pain in the birth.

The Leboyer method of childbirth does not focus on pain management for the mother; rather, it emphasizes the extreme sensitivity of the newborn. According to Frederick Leboyer, who developed the approach, the delivery environment should consist of dim lighting and little noise. Following minimal handling, the newborn should be immediately immersed in warm water. While this approach was popular in the seventies, today few hospitals practice the Leboyer method due to difficulties encountered, such as not recognizing newborn problems due to the darkness of the delivery room. Some of its positive aspects, however, have been incorporated into other programs.

Many options are open to you. Not everyone can utilize Lamaze successfully. On the other hand, not everyone has difficult or painful labors. The important point is that, within limits, you can choose from many methods of making the labor and delivery a wonderful experience. You should remember, however, that a situation may arise during delivery — perhaps the baby is too big for the pelvis, or there is fetal distress — which requires a cesarean section. Discussing this possibility with your Lamaze instructor or your physician will help prepare you for this eventuality so that you will know what to expect.

Electronic Fetal Monitoring

During labor, your baby's heart rate must be checked from time to time to assure that there is no fetal distress. This may be done by listening through the mother's abdomen with a special stethoscope or Doppler instrument. Alternatively, the fetal heart may be monitored electronically by a device strapped to the maternal abdomen; this is safe and painless. After the fetal membranes are ruptured, the baby's heart may be more directly monitored by placing an electrode on its scalp. The advantage of electronic fetal monitoring (EFM) is that it will provide continuous surveillance.

In low-risk pregnancies, there is no proof that continuous EFM is superior to intermittent listening to the fetal heart (every fifteen minutes in the first stage of labor). However, in pregnancies with risk factors, there is no argument: EFM is essential and can prevent severe undetected hypoxic (lack of oxygen) episodes to the fetus. The key is to remember your goal — to have a healthy baby. But since choices in clinical medicine are not always clearcut, the best advice is to ask your doctor what is recommended in your situation.

Rooming-in

Many hospitals offer programs in which the baby stays with the mother in her room around the clock. There are many advantages to this rooming-in arrangement. The mother is with her baby continuously to establish closeness and bonding. In addition, the mother learns to take care of the baby totally during the first few days of life. There are no periods of separation.

Non-rooming-in routines entail having the baby brought to the mother's room five or six times during each twenty-four-hour period for feeding and caressing. At the end of each session, the baby is returned to the nursery. This certainly affords more rest for the mother. But it also means that the mother may experience feelings of separation. It may be difficult to predict your needs beforehand.

Some hospitals offer programs in which the mother can

have rooming-in during the daytime, but the baby goes to the nursery overnight. Of course, the baby is brought back to the mother for the 2:00 A.M. feeding! This really offers the best of both worlds for the mother — maximizing newborn contact in the day and rest at night. Many women prefer this option since they realize that once they are home they will not experience this luxury again anytime soon.

Breast-feeding

The choice between breast-feeding and bottle-feeding is very important. Breast-feeding can be a magnificently intimate time. It also provides your newborn with a nutritionally balanced beginning. The breasts' initial secretion, colostrum, contains antibodies not found in formula which bolster the newborn's immune responses. While breast-feeding definitely allows for bonding, it may also help to prevent infections, allergies, and obesity in the newborn.

Many women with career and work restrictions are concerned that breast-feeding is not an option for them because they must return to work. It is really not an all-or-nothing decision. You may miss a very rewarding experience if you view breast-feeding this way. Ideally, breast-feeding is done for many months, but you can breast-feed your newborn baby for much shorter periods of time, if that is your best or only option. Some mothers are able to pump their breasts to have breast milk available for bottle-feeding when they resume work. Alternatively, mothers can fully breast-feed for whatever time they have off and then start supplementing with bottle-feeding when they go back to their jobs. La Leche League International is a valuable resource for breast-feeding information.

Totally breast-fed infants may refuse to take a bottle. Exposing the breast-fed newborn to the bottle can save a lot of headaches later on. Knowing her baby will accept an occasional bottle-feeding gives the mother the freedom to be away during feeding time once in a while, as well as the option of bottle-feeding when or where breast-feeding may be inconvenient or difficult. In addition, bottle-feeding gives the father a chance for intimacy with the newborn and for shared feeding responsibility.

Choosing a Pediatrician

Your choice of pediatrician is vital. Pediatricians are often members of the delivery team and perform the initial evaluation of your newborn. Well before delivery, you should gather recommendations from friends and health professionals. Just as you carefully select the health professional who delivers your child, it is best to pick a pediatrician you really trust.

Your first pediatric visit will be approximately two weeks postpartum. Take this opportunity not only to address questions you may have regarding your child's well-being but also to allay any doubts you may have about breast-feeding, parenting, or whatever!

Child Care

You will be contemplating the management and balance of work out of the home with your new responsibilities in the home. Begin planning for child care early. Whether you plan to use in-home child care, family day care, or the services of a day care center, before delivering, develop a resource list of baby-sitters, day care centers (near home *and* work), and support persons. Interview prospective caregivers. Visit facilities during hours of operation, inquiring about the program schedule, flexibility, costs, group size, and staff training. Determine who uses the services and if they are satisfied. Learn about all the alternatives. Parenthood presents many options and rewards. The choices you make can enhance your enjoyment of the profound adventure you are sharing.

[4]

Finances
Theda L. Marinelli, B.S.

Having a baby can be such a delightful event. But even something so wonderful has a downside: it costs a lot of money! The consolation is that if you are planning to have a baby, you have time on your side. You can, therefore, do some creative financial planning.

IN ADDITION to preparing yourself physically and emotionally for a child, preparing yourself financially is important. The birth of your baby should be a happy occasion and should not be clouded by large unpaid or unexpected medical bills.

Investigating the costs you are likely to incur, the kinds of payment arrangements that can be made, and how much of the expense will be covered by insurance will help you avoid unnecessary worry. The following pages offer an overview to assist you in determining your financial liability for your obstetric care.

What Types of Bills Can I Expect to Receive?

The bills that you can expect to receive for your pregnancy care will fall into three main categories: obstetric care, ancillary services, and hospitalization. Although it is possible to provide general information on those services and fees, actual policies and procedures vary not only from area to area but from office to office.

Obstetric Care

Most offices now bill for what is called "total OB care and delivery" or "global care." This fee will include all of your prenatal visits in the office and the delivery itself. It is based upon the type of care you are expected to require. The determining factors are whether or not your care is routine or high risk and whether you have a vaginal or cesarean delivery. While the type of care you are expected to require can generally be estimated at the time of your first obstetrical visit, you can expect the actual charges to vary from the originally quoted fee if your medical situation changes.

Ancillary Services

Ancillary services are any services that are performed in addition to the global care mentioned above. They may be rendered by your obstetrician or by another provider. Different patients require different levels of ancillary services; the number and type of services you require will be determined by your obstetrician and your medical situation. Some of these may include:

Laboratory services. At a minimum, you will have a complete prenatal laboratory workup done at the time of your first visit unless it was already done in preparation for pregnancy. Other laboratory tests may be ordered during the course of your pregnancy if required for your medical management.

Prenatal testing services. The most common prenatal testing services are ultrasound (sonogram), nonstress testing, and chorionic villus sampling or amniocentesis. These may be required to assess the health and development of the fetus.

Prenatal medical and surgical services. These services may be necessary if your medical condition requires medical or surgical care that extends beyond the scope of routine prenatal care. This may include hospitalization or a surgical procedure.

Anesthesia. Often, during the course of labor and delivery, a patient may require pain relief. An anesthesiologist may be asked to place an epidural anesthetic or give a general anesthetic for delivery.

Pathology. Occasionally, your obstetrician may find something unusual about the placenta. He or she may, therefore, ask a pathologist to examine it for further evaluation.

Pediatrics. Most hospitals will have a pediatrician examine the infant prior to discharge for general health assessment. Additional pediatric services may also be necessary at the time of delivery.

Hospital Fees

Your hospital bill will include room charges and services provided by hospital personnel and departments during the course of your stay. Since it usually does not include fees for the services provided by physicians, you can expect to receive separate bills from the physician and the hospital.

How Will These Bills Be Paid?

Most patients do not consider how they will pay for pregnancy care until after they have become pregnant. Unfortunately, that may be too late. Some insurance policies do not cover obstetric care at all, while some cover it only in specific situations or only when care is provided by certain physicians. The time to thoroughly research your insurance coverage is when you are considering a pregnancy. In that way, you can make necessary adjustments to your coverage or rearrange your budget beforehand.

Whether or not you have insurance coverage, it is important to find out what the expected fees are for all anticipated services, and to learn the payment policies and procedures for each of the offices. The net effect of insurance coverage is to reduce your personal financial liability for these services. However, it does not determine the method and timing of your payments. This is established by the particular office billing for the service.

You should talk to the billing personnel in your obstetrician's office as early as possible. They will be able to provide you with most, if not all, of the information that you need on fees and payment arrangements. However, it is also good policy to talk directly to billing personnel in the hospital and other offices from which you expect to receive bills. When you select your obstetrician and hospital these questions may be helpful:

- What is the fee for prenatal visits and delivery? What specific services are included in that fee?
- How will the fee change if I should require a cesarean section or if my pregnancy becomes high risk?
- What ancillary services are provided and billed for by the obstetrician?
- What are the policies and procedures for payment for my care?
- What are the fees, payment arrangements, and phone numbers for billing personnel for any ancillary and hospital services that may be required?

If you have a "secondary" insurance policy (see below), you should ask the following question:

• What is the policy for submitting secondary insurance claims? Does the office submit the claim for direct payment? Am I required to pay that balance and then submit for reimbursement?

These additional questions should be asked if your insurance carrier "contracts" with physicians, as explained below:

• Does the physician "contract" or "participate" with my insurance carrier?
• Am I required to obtain an authorized referral from my primary-care physician in order for services to be covered?

It will also be helpful to ask the following questions of your hospital's billing personnel:

• What is the estimated fee for my hospital stay?
• What is the estimated fee for my baby's hospital stay?
• What is the labor and delivery room rate? The nursery rate?
• What are the usual components of the estimated fee?
• What are the policies and procedures for insurance submission and payment?

The total fee for all components of your care will vary greatly depending upon the area in which you live, due primarily to differences in malpractice premiums and the cost of doing business in that area. Data for 1987 from the Health Insurance Association of America gives these cost estimates as a national average:

	Vaginal Birth*	Cesarean Birth*
Rural area	$2,340	$4,040
Urban area	$2,800	$4,450

* Includes hospital and professional fees. Does not include anesthesia ($60 average) or pediatric newborn exam ($86 average).

Costs in major cities may well exceed these averages, which may also vary based on the level of care and length of hospitalization you or the baby may require. This only serves to emphasize the importance of determining as many of the costs as you can and the extent of your insurance coverage before you become pregnant.

Three general kinds of arrangements are typically made to cover payment of fees for total OB care and delivery. The same types of arrangements will generally apply to other services that are provided. You should be aware that only an estimated fee can be provided to you until you actually deliver. Therefore, in the case of prepayment arrangements, there may still be a balance due from you after delivery.

Full payment prior to delivery. Some offices will require that the entire estimated fee be paid prior to delivery. Although this is less frequent for insured patients, it will almost always apply to uninsured, or "self-pay," patients.

Prepayment of estimated liability. Generally, your insurance will not cover the full cost of your obstetric care. In this instance, many offices will calculate the estimated insurance payment amount and use that figure to determine your estimated liability. You will then be asked to pay this portion prior to delivery. This is the most common practice for the global fee.

Payment of residual balance only. In some instances, you will only be billed after the insurance payment has been received. This is becoming more infrequent.

Insurance: What Are the Different Types?

Before we begin any discussion of types of insurance policies, it is useful to be familiar with the following terms:

Deductible. The "first dollars" of charges incurred within a given year (usually a calendar year). The patient is entirely responsible for payment of this amount, and the insurance benefits do not start to apply until this amount has been exceeded.

Copayment. The percentage or dollar amount of each charge for which the patient is responsible. Many policies will only pay a percentage or set amount for each service, and the patient is responsible for payment of the balance. In the case of managed-care plans (see below), this copayment may be a specific dollar amount for each visit or type of service, and payment of this amount is generally required at the time of the visit.

Primary and secondary coverage. If a patient is covered by more than one policy (e.g., the wife has her own insurance and is also covered by the husband's), one will be primary (billed first) and one will be secondary (billed for any balance not covered by the primary). In the vast majority of the cases, the patient's insurance is the primary and any other insurance coverage is the secondary. This has two notable exceptions. First, if one person has two policies, one will normally cover only hospital-provided services and the other will cover all physician services. Second, if both parents have insurance covering the child, the only way to accurately determine the primary is to contact the insurance carriers directly. Some localities use a date-of-birth rule to determine primary and some do not.

Contracting or participating physician. A physician who has a specified contract with an insurance carrier. If your plan offers contracts to physicians and you use a noncontracting physician, benefits may be reduced, your copayment amount may increase, or services may not be covered at all. Not all insurance companies offer such contracts to physicians.

Accepts assignment. This applies to insurance carriers that do not offer contracts to physicians (currently the majority of traditional fee-for-service plans do not). If a physician accepts assignment, it means that the insurance company will make payment directly to the physician. There is no effect on your out-of-pocket expense.

Precertification and/or length-of-stay determination. An increasing number of insurance carriers now require that preauthorization be obtained for any hospital stay. Failure to obtain this may result in either a denial of payment or a significant reduction in payment from the insurance carrier. In addition, coverage may be limited to a specific number of hospital days.

UCR (usual, customary, and reasonable). Most insurance companies now have a maximum amount that they will pay for a specific service. This is called the UCR amount and is generally based on some percentage of average charges for a given area. Your physician's fee may be above or below this maximum amount because of local variations in malpractice premiums and other business costs or because of the geographic area or the method used by the insurance company to make its calculations.

Primary-care physician. Under HMO or some managed-care coverage, the physician who is responsible for your primary care, and for authorizing your referral (and therefore payment) to other providers of medical care. Depending on the type of plan, this may or may not be your obstetrician.

There are hundreds of different types of insurance policies currently available. While each policy differs in its specifics, it will generally fall into one of the following categories.

Traditional fee-for-service (also called indemnity coverage). This type of insurance can be used at any office or facility and provides reimbursement for each service rendered. The reimbursement rate will generally vary based on the type of service (e.g., physician, laboratory, hospital). In the majority of cases there will be some out-of-pocket expenses, either in the form of a deductible or a copayment.

With this type of insurance, you will generally receive

bills for the services as they are rendered and payment will be made under one of the payment arrangements mentioned above.

Health Maintenance Organization (HMO). This type of insurance requires that all of your care be provided by the HMO and its contracting physicians and hospitals (except in emergency situations) in order for the services to be covered. Thus, your choice of physicians is generally limited to those contracted with by the HMO in order for the services to be covered.

With this type of coverage, the HMO is billed directly and you will generally not receive any bills for your care, unless certain services are excluded under your policy or your plan requires a copayment amount.

Managed-care plans — IPAs (independent practice associations) and PPOs (preferred provider organizations). These plans are a hybrid of traditional fee-for-service insurance and the coverage provided by the HMO. Choice of physicians and hospitals is generally limited to contracting members of the IPA or PPO, via an authorized referral from your primary-care physician. A significant reduction in benefits will generally apply if a noncontracting physician is used. For some plans, deductibles and copayments are also in effect.

With this type of insurance, you may or may not receive bills for a portion of your care. Again, this will generally be for services that are excluded under your coverage or for any applicable copayment or deductible amounts.

What Does My Insurance Cover?

The only way to determine what your insurance covers, and at what rate, is to ask. And the only sources of precise information are either the insurance company itself, your insurance agent, or the insurance benefits coordinator at your place of employment. While your physician's office may have general information on your insurance company, it will not have specific information about the particular contract between you and your insurance company. Here are some suggested questions to ask your insurance representative:

- Does my policy cover only physician services, only hospital services, or both?
- Is obstetrical care covered? Does the policy cover routine pregnancy care or does it cover only complications?
- Based upon the specific date of my enrollment under this policy, is there any waiting period before obstetrical care is covered? (Many policies have a "preexisting condition" clause that precludes coverage for pregnancy care if you were pregnant at the time of enrollment or became pregnant shortly prior to or after enrollment.)
- Am I limited to certain physicians and hospitals in order for benefits to be paid? How much will benefits be reduced if I use a noncontracting physician or hospital?
- Does my plan require that an authorized referral be provided by my primary-care physician in order for services to be covered?
- Does my plan require precertification to be obtained in order for services to be covered? Is there a separate certification for physician versus hospital services? At what point must this be done? What forms are required? What is the normal length of stay that is authorized?
- Will you accept a claim for total OB care and delivery, or must each visit and the delivery be billed separately?
- What forms are required for submitting a claim for services? Can the standard HCFA 1500 or UB82 forms (rather than company forms) be used for the physician? For the hospital? What is the exact address to which claims should be mailed?

- (If you currently have individual coverage only:) Can I change to family coverage? If so, will the baby be covered at birth or will there be a waiting period?
- (If you have family coverage:) At what point is the baby covered? Is routine newborn care covered? Is "well baby" care covered? What forms must be completed, and when, to ensure that my baby has continuous coverage from birth?
- If both parents have insurance policies that cover the child, which is primary?
- Does the policy have a maximum total dollar benefit? (Some policies will only pay a set dollar amount, regardless of the total charges.)
- How are benefits calculated for the following categories of services? Are payments made as a percentage of the total charge or as a set fee per service? Is there any applicable deductible amount? What is my copayment for each type of service?
  prenatal care and delivery
  laboratory tests
  prenatal tests
  pathology tests
  anesthesia services
  pediatric services
  circumcision
  other physician medical and surgical services
  hospital-generated charges: room and board; labor and delivery room; nursery, regular or intensive care; laboratory, medications, supplies, etc.; nursing care

What if I Have No Insurance or if I Change Policies During the Course of My Pregnancy?

If you have no insurance coverage for your obstetric care, payment for all services will be your responsibility. Talk to the billing personnel in all offices from which you expect to receive services. Ask specifically about deposit requirements or available payment arrangements. Some hospitals and clinics will offer reduced fees to uninsured patients. One important note is that, while cost should be a consideration, it should not be the only factor in choosing where to receive your medical care.

A change in insurance coverage while you are pregnant could mean that further obstetrical services will not be covered by the new insurance company. It could also mean that you are required to use the services of a contracting physician in order to receive benefits. In this instance, it becomes imperative to contact the new insurance company to determine the extent of your coverage and whether or not services performed by your current obstetrician will be covered. The questions listed above should be asked of the new company.

This chapter has provided some answers but many more questions. That was its intent. Each patient's financial and insurance situation is different, and there is no one answer to the question "How much will this pregnancy cost and how will it be paid for?" In addition, the insurance industry's policies and procedures are constantly changing in an effort to contain costs and respond to changing health care patterns. Specific information that is valid today will be outdated tomorrow. Therefore, the importance of obtaining specific answers to all of your questions cannot be overemphasized. We are all consumers of the insurance company "product." We should know what we have purchased and how it is to be used.

By asking the questions presented here, you will be better able to determine and structure the required financial resources, so that when your child is born the only question left to ask will be "Isn't the baby adorable?"

[PART II]

The Gift of Life

[5]

The Menstrual Cycle, Fertility, and Infertility
Michael J. Zinaman, M.D.

Throughout history, the menstrual cycle has been considered one of the great mysteries of life. And today, when the majority of hormonal events that lead to normal menses are known, it seems even more amazing that many women have clocklike cycles. For example, the occurrence of ovulation is almost always fourteen days before menstruation.

In this chapter, Dr. Zinaman presents the basic physiology of the menstrual cycle. In addition, you will learn how to determine the time of ovulation, information that is extremely important if you are trying to conceive. This helps you to become pregnant or to avoid pregnancy when the situation is not favorable — for instance, if you have developed a viral illness. Not everyone is quite so fortunate as to be able to achieve a pregnancy at will. Indeed, many couples find that they are unsuccessful after one or more years of attempting it. These couples may have one or more of a number of problems that can lead to infertility. In the past, infertility was considered to be primarily the fault of the woman, but today we realize this is neither fair nor correct. The causes of infertility are probably more closely distributed between both partners, as will be outlined in this chapter. In fact, as we learn more about male fertility we realize the increasing importance of these factors. If a couple has difficulty conceiving, it is very important to get professional help, because approximately 90 percent of couples will still achieve a pregnancy if they undergo therapy. Probably the best rule of thumb is to recognize the problem early. Diagnosis and therapy can then be initiated to minimize the considerable discouragement and emotional factors associated with infertility.

Over the last few decades, couples have strived to gain control over their childbearing plans. The widespread availability and use of reliable means of contraception has made this possible. Perhaps the most important reason couples today actively plan their families is the rise of women in the work force. Women are contributing more than ever to their family's economic prosperity, and many have reached a point where career choices are dictating the *best* timing for having children. The natural consequence has been a change in the age at which women are having their first child.

With women delaying childbearing, there has been an increase in awareness of the possible adverse consequences this may have on their fertility. Many research studies demonstrate increased fertility-related problems experienced by women who have chosen to delay having a family.

This chapter deals with the physiology of the normal menstrual cycle, our knowledge about the relative fertile times of the cycle, signs and symptoms women have that reflect their fertile period, and the probability of conception occurring in a given cycle. It also reviews general infertility considerations.

The Menstrual Cycle

The menstrual cycle is a very complex process that requires active input from the brain (hypothalamus), pituitary

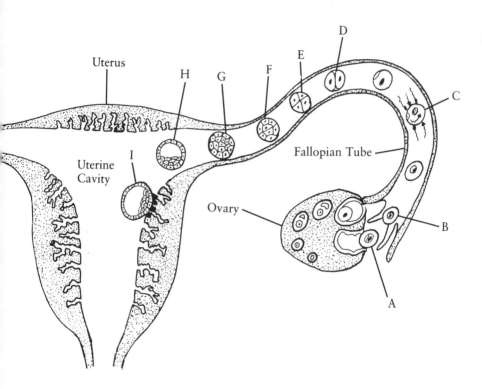

Figure 5-1. Normal Fertilization. The process of conception begins when the egg is released from the ovarian follicle at ovulation (A). It enters the end of the fallopian tube (B). Fertilization occurs when an active sperm penetrates the ovum (C). Only one sperm enters the ovum; the others are blocked on the surface. The fertilized egg then divides and grows (D–G), remaining in the fallopian tube for a few days before reaching the uterine cavity. Approximately seventy-two hours after fertilization, the embryo can be found in the uterine cavity (H). One to two days later, the embryo burrows into the uterine lining and implantation takes place (I). It is shortly after this process that pregnancy hormone produced by the embryo reaches the mother's circulating blood. The embryo then grows with one part forming the placenta and the other the developing fetus.

gland, ovaries, and uterus. The normal menstrual cycle is defined as lasting anywhere from twenty-three to thirty-five days. While this is a rather broad definition of normal, most women have cycles that vary from twenty-six to thirty-one days. Indeed, many are extremely regular, varying by only one or two days per month. This reflects the highly tuned system at work in the female body.

To facilitate discussion about the menstrual cycle, physicians have arbitrarily designated the first day of menstrual bleeding as day number one of the cycle. The last day of the cycle is the day before the first day of the next menstrual cycle.

The menstrual cycle is composed of two phases. The first is the follicular phase, which begins on day one of the cycle and continues up to and including ovulation (release of the egg from the ovary), about midway through the cycle. This phase is initiated by the release of follicle-stimulating hormone (FSH), which causes the growth of several follicles, cells in the ovary that surround immature eggs. Usually, only one egg will ripen each month. As the follicle grows, the ovaries release increasing levels of the hormone estrogen. The estrogen, in turn, causes growth of the lining of the uterus. When the egg is mature, the follicle sends a message (estrogen) to the pituitary gland, causing a tremendous release of LH (luteinizing hormone). About thirty-four hours afterward, the follicle ruptures and releases the egg into the fallopian tube. It is the great rise in the level of the hormone LH that serves as the basis for many of the home tests to detect ovulation which are sold nationwide. It is useful to know that with every menstrual cycle, a woman develops an ovarian cyst that can reach one inch in diameter. Therefore, the finding on exam of a small ovarian cyst is usually a normal event. It usually disappears by the end of the cycle or shortly thereafter.

Following the release of the egg, the ruptured follicle fills with blood and becomes a yellow mass called the corpus luteum (literally, "yellow body"). Hence the name luteal phase for the second part of the cycle. The corpus luteum secretes estrogen as well as large amounts of progesterone. The progesterone prepares the lining of the uterus for implantation of the embryo should conception occur. If implantation does not occur, the corpus luteum begins to regress after fourteen days, with declining progesterone production. This basically means that in the absence of conception, the second half of the menstrual cycle (after ovulation) is of a rather fixed length. Indeed, the majority of the variation in cycle length occurs in the first half, or follicular phase, of the cycle. The drop in circulating progesterone has its effect by withdrawing support for the lining of the uterus. The next menstrual cycle is ushered in as menses begins and the old uterine lining is shed in preparation for a new growth later in the cycle.

The Egg and Sperm

Before one can talk specifically about women's relative fertile times during the menstrual cycle, a review of our knowledge of egg and sperm survival is needed. The egg is released from the ovary about thirty-four to thirty-six hours after the onset of the LH surge that comes from the pituitary gland. It is normally picked up by the fallopian tube, where fertilization takes place. Epidemiologic studies as well as knowledge gained from recent in vitro (test-tube) fertilization studies suggest that the egg remains capable of being fertilized for a rather short period of time. In fact, most scientists believe this period to be somewhat less than twenty-four hours and perhaps even less than twelve. This leaves us with a remarkably brief time span in which conception can occur.

Studies on the functional survival of sperm in the female have shown their ability to survive and fertilize for rather prolonged periods. The female cervix produces mucus under the influence of estrogen. The mucus appears to play a nourishing role for the sperm and allows them to remain in this "reservoir" for as long as four to five days. Under normal conditions, there is a steady release of sperm from the cervical mucus. They swim up through the uterine cavity and into the fallopian tubes. In this manner, the sperm can be waiting for the egg for several days after a single act of intercourse. One could then say that the sperm's ability to survive for several days compensates for the short life span of the egg.

There have been claims made recently that older sperm (those resulting from intercourse several days prior to ovulation) are more likely to carry a Y chromosome, which would then result in a pregnancy with the delivery of a male infant. But, carefully executed scientific studies do not validate these claims.

Cyclical Symptoms of Ovulation

Women frequently have recognizable signs and symptoms during the menstrual cycle that indicate when ovulation is occurring. By learning how to interpret these signs, you can optimize your chance of achieving pregnancy in a given cycle.

Cervical mucus is a product of the uterine cervix; its production and consistency are under the influence of the ovarian hormones estrogen and progesterone. During the follicular phase of the cycle, estrogen levels are rising as the follicle with its egg grows and matures. The cervix responds to estrogen with a progressive increase in mucus production. In addition, the mucus becomes thinner, more watery in consistency, and clear. A long-noted characteristic of fertile mucus is called *spinnbarkeit*. This refers to the stretchability of the mucus, and it too increases with estrogen. The thinner, more stretchable mucus makes it easier for sperm to enter the uterus. As the estrogen reaches its peak, the woman is usually aware of an increased discharge at the entrance to the vagina. This is due to the mucus coming from the cervix. Occasionally, she may interpret this discharge as representing a vaginal infection, but it can easily be differentiated from infection by the lack of foul odor and the absence of itching or burning, as well as by its cyclical nature.

The estrogen peak also has the effect of inducing the pituitary gland to release large amounts of LH (the LH surge). This then results in ovulation. Thus, if a woman is aware of the temporal change of events, she can use her cervical mucus as an index of fertility. Studies have clearly shown that peak mucus activity is followed by ovulation in about twenty-four to thirty-six hours. Intercourse can then be planned around this time to maximize the chances of conception.

Several other events commonly occur around the time of ovulation and indicate a high level of fertility. The first is a sensation experienced by many women called *mittelschmerz*. This refers to pain in the pelvic area derived from the follicle that is about to or has just ruptured to release the egg. It is thought to be due to a small amount of blood and other substances that come from the follicle. The pain is one-sided and has been reported to be either sharp or dull and achy in nature. It usually lasts about twenty-four hours.

Other signs and symptoms such as bloating, breast tenderness, and light spotting occur around the time of ovulation. If a woman exercises a high degree of self-awareness, she can frequently pinpoint her ovulation to within a twenty-four-hour time span.

Women have at their disposal two other relatively accurate methods to determine retrospectively when they ovulate. A woman who has a very regular menstrual cycle can thus use one of these methods to predict the times when intercourse is most likely to result in pregnancy. The simplest of these relates to the fact that the second part (luteal phase) of the menstrual cycle is of a relatively fixed duration. The number of days from ovulation to the last day of the cycle is around fourteen. After the occurrence of menses, one may count back fourteen days into the previous cycle and attempt to pinpoint ovulation. For many women, this is an accurate method to determine if they had intercourse around the time of ovulation.

The second method entails daily measurement of the basal body temperature. This refers to taking one's temperature upon awakening in the morning and prior to getting out of bed. Special thermometers are available that allow accurate readings to the nearest tenth of a degree. The underlying mechanism behind this method is as follows: As mentioned earlier in the chapter, progesterone is produced by the corpus luteum soon after ovulation. Progesterone itself has the ability to reset the brain's thermostat approximately one-half to one degree Fahrenheit higher. If a woman takes and records her basal temperature each day, she will note that about midway through her cycle her temperature rises by a half degree or more and remains at that level until the end of the cycle, at which time it drops to its earlier level. For the most part, ovulation generally occurs about twenty-four hours prior to the first day of sustained temperature elevation. Elevations, while not great in magnitude, can usually be seen without difficulty if plotted on appropriate graph paper. Most studies suggest that as many as 90 percent of ovulatory cycles will show this typical temperature pattern, which is tied to the two menstrual phases.

If a woman has been using oral contraceptives, then once she discontinues their use, she must wait for the hormones to wear off and for her body to resume its natural cycles prior to attaining pregnancy. The time required may range from a few weeks up to three months. If the delay in resuming cycles is longer, it should be brought to the attention of the physician. Pregnancy can occur prior to the resumption of menses. If this happens, the time of ovulation may be uncertain and sonography may be necessary to determine the date of gestation. Becoming pregnant immediately after stopping oral contraceptives does not increase the risk of abortion or congenital malformations.

Infertility

The ability to conceive is dependent upon frequent successful intercourse. Deposition of sperm deep in the vagina allows them to gain entrance into the cervix and subsequently the fallopian tubes, where fertilization takes place. Even though the timing of intercourse may coincide with ovulation, there is only about a 30 percent chance that pregnancy will result in any given cycle. This is important to remember so that couples do not become concerned after one or two months of what appeared to be well-timed intercourse. Most authorities agree that couples who have intercourse on two spaced occasions weekly will demonstrate normal fertility. A slight increase in the conception rate per cycle does occur if more frequent intercourse is practiced. Despite this, there is no benefit to having intercourse more than every other day, since sperm counts can drop dramatically. In the same vein, "saving it up" for the right time is also of no benefit: sperm numbers may increase but performance parameters such as sperm motion do not, and conception rates have not been shown to increase.

Infertility, by the most strict definition, refers to a couple's inability to conceive following one year of unprotected intercourse. This obviously assumes that the couple is having frequent and successful intercourse. This has very little to do with sexual gratification and satisfaction, but rather with sperm being in the right place at the right time. In addition, infertility can be categorized as primary (the couple has no history of a previous pregnancy) or secondary (previous pregnancy, regardless of outcome).

By most available estimates, infertility affects about 15 percent of couples today. Approximately 60 percent to 70 percent of couples will achieve a pregnancy in the first three months of trying. Another 10 percent or so will be successful within six months, and an additional 5 percent in one year. A few additional percent will be successful during the second year. This leaves us with approximately 15 percent who will seek professional advice.

Causes of Infertility

The general causes of infertility are listed in Table 5-1. As noted, the pelvic factor in females accounts for 30 to 50 percent of cases. This includes two of the more common disease entities that affect a woman's fertility. The first is endometriosis, a condition whereby tissue resembling the lining of the uterus implants in the pelvic cavity and undergoes cyclic growth and bleeding much like the true lining does. Considerable scarring and anatomic deformity may result, causing occlusion of the fallopian tubes or affecting their ability to pick up the egg. The second condition results from pelvic inflammatory disease (PID), which is infection

Table 5-1 CAUSES OF INFERTILITY	
Pelvic pathology	30–50%
Cervical hostility	5–25%
Male factor	25–40%
Ovulation defect	15–25%
Unknown cause	10–20%

and inflammation of uterus, tubes, and ovaries. Episodes of PID can cause considerable and often irreversible destruction of the reproductive organs. The infectious bacteria gonorrhea and chlamydia are responsible for the vast majority of pelvic inflammatory disease cases in the United States.

Ovulatory disorders represent 15 to 25 percent of the instances of infertility. These may manifest themselves as a history of infrequent or no ovulation. With what we know about the brief life span of eggs, we can easily imagine difficulty in conceiving if only two or three are released in a year. Hormonal imbalances of numerous glands in the body frequently play a role in defects of ovulation.

When the fallopian tubes have been severely damaged from either endometriosis or infection, the couple has as a last resort in vitro fertilization. This process involves the operative removal of eggs from the ovary and their placement directly with sperm in a dish in the laboratory. After fertilization, the developing embryo is placed in the uterus via the cervix. The fallopian tubes are bypassed completely.

The so-called male factor is recognized today as being one of the more important causes of a couple's inability to achieve a pregnancy. This generally refers to sperm problems but may also relate to failure of ejaculation or retrograde ejaculation (into the bladder). Indeed, the infertility rate attributed to men has more than doubled in the last ten years. This is not so much due to a change in the men themselves as it is due to our increased understanding of problems with sperm physiology. In the majority of cases in which a lower than optimal sperm count is believed to play a role in a couple's infertility, the hormonal parameters and physical characteristics of the men are no different from those of men with proven fertility.

Other factors such as cervical mucus problems and a

variety of other disorders may also be found to contribute to a couple's diminished fertility potential. Cervical mucus problems can range from failure to make any (after surgery on the cervix) to frank hostility, in which the mucus contains antibodies that kill the sperm.

Despite the most sophisticated testing available to date, a small percentage of couples will be unable to conceive without any apparent reason. A relatively recent treatment called gamete intrafallopian tube transfer (GIFT) has been successful in many of these couples. The egg and sperm are placed together in the fallopian tube, where fertilization can then take place.

At this point, it is important to stress that frequently both the female and the male will demonstrate factors that contribute to the overall diminished fertility potential. A methodical approach to correcting these factors will better the chances of conception. In many cases it is not possible to place the "blame" on one person or the other as the primary cause of infertility.

Age and Fertility

Another topic that has received increased interest in the last few years is the role of age in infertility. For a variety of reasons, the woman's increasingly important role in the workplace being the most often cited, physicians have noted a postponement in the starting of families. With this trend came an apparent increase in fertility problems. This observation generated considerable interest and several studies by investigators. What has been found is as follows: Women in the 21-to-25 and 26-30 age groups demonstrate normal fertility potential (25 to 30 percent per cycle). In the 31-35 age group, there is a trend toward a lower conception rate (20 to 25 percent per cycle). This group can probably achieve the same overall conception rate, but it seems to take somewhat longer to do so. In women over the age of 35, a significant decline in fertility potential is evident. As many as 50 percent of women in this age category will have major problems achieving a pregnancy, and they make up a disproportionate percentage of the patients visiting infertility specialists.

Seeking Help

One very important question often raised refers to when a couple should be concerned about their ability to have children. While no rigid guidelines can be uniformly applied to all couples, there are several that can be useful in a general fashion. If you recall, about 75 percent of those who are going to conceive do so in the first six months of trying. Failure at this point would be reason for concern, and use of any number of methods previously discussed to ensure adequate intercourse during the fertile period is warranted. If the woman is in the upper age range, a visit to a specialist is also appropriate at this time. Other factors such as irregular menses or a history of previous pelvic infections or endometriosis would also suggest a visit to a specialist. Previous abdominal surgery, most commonly for the removal of an appendix (especially if it was ruptured), may have caused scarring and distortion of the normal pelvic anatomy and may serve as a warning for potential fertility-related problems. While the list of possible historical factors that may have contributed to a reduced ability to conceive is rather long, making use of the signs and symptoms of the woman's fertile period could, with adequate intercourse practices, generally result in conception over a six-to-twelve-month time span.

In this chapter, we have laid the foundation for increasing our understanding of the underlying reproductive physiology of the female. By being aware of her menstrual cycle's follicular phase, with rising estrogen levels, and luteal phase, with rising estrogen and progesterone levels, a woman can use a variety of simple and inexpensive methods to identify her most fertile period.

Once they understand the survival patterns of eggs and sperm, couples can also time their intercourse patterns during the fertile period to maximize their chances of achieving a pregnancy. In addition, couples should now be better able to recognize potential problems if conception does not occur. The ability to have children is for most couples a very special part of their relationship, and it is through education that they can actively play a part in understanding their respective roles.

[6]

Mother and Fetus: Changing, Growing
Kimberly K. Leslie, M.D.

In order for the mother's body to accommodate a growing fetus, some profound changes must take place. Many of these adjustments can be recognized by the mother as changes in appearance or sensations, while others are "silent" and occur without the mother's knowledge or awareness. For instance, increased frequency of urination and increased size and tenderness of the breasts are early signs of pregnancy caused by changes in the maternal physiology. A less discernible change essential to the well-being of the fetus is the increase in the total volume of blood within the mother's circulatory system. Her heart rate rises slightly and the amount of blood pumped per minute by her heart increases considerably. These are just a few examples of the many ways the mother's body changes to support the developing fetus.

In this chapter, Dr. Leslie presents an overview of maternal and fetal physiology during pregnancy. Reading this section will give you a basic understanding of how mother and fetus adapt during gestation.

I N A MEDICAL SENSE, the study of human physiology is the study of the vital functions and processes of the body. Physiology as it relates to pregnancy is the study of the functional changes the mother and fetus undergo as the pregnancy progresses. The first part of this chapter will be devoted to a discussion of the physiologic adaptations of the mother to pregnancy. The remaining two parts of the chapter will focus on the fetus and the placenta.

The study of the physiology of pregnancy is of particular importance for an understanding of the benefits of preconception planning. By knowing the functional and developmental stages of the fetus, you will have a better understanding of when the fetus is especially vulnerable to teratogens (agents capable of causing fetal damage) and drugs. The study of the maternal physiologic adaptations to pregnancy will help you to assess the importance of adequate nutrition and of prepregnancy cardiovascular and muscular fitness.

It is especially comforting to know that the changes described are normal and expected. They allow for the safe coexistence of you and your baby during the pregnancy, and return your body to its prepregnancy condition within several weeks after birth.

The Mother and Her Adaptation to Pregnancy

How the mother conceives, nourishes, and fosters the growth of an immunologically foreign being, the fetus, inside her own body remains one of the great mysteries of science. She adapts to the growth of her "passenger" in many amazing ways, providing the fetus with oxygen, all of the vital nutrients and foodstuffs for life and growth, and a waste-removal system designed to clear the fetal blood of carbon dioxide and other by-products. All of this occurs in a safe, warm, and sterile environment, the uterus, from which, under the usual conditions, the infant is expelled only when mature enough to function in the world as a separate individual.

For the mother, pregnancy is a state of increased demand on all body functions. Essentially every organ is affected, including the cardiovascular, respiratory, urinary, endocrine, musculoskeletal, digestive, metabolic, and, most especially, the reproductive systems. The majority of changes are attributable either to the rapid enlargement of the uterus to accommodate the growing fetus or to the hormonal changes that accompany pregnancy. The hormones estrogen and progesterone are greatly increased in pregnancy and have many important effects on all body systems. By occupying ever-increasing space, the pregnant uterus causes changes in other organs. This may cause some discomforts for the mother.

For example, the growth of the uterus causes stretching of the ligaments that run from the pelvic sidewalls to the top of the uterus on both sides. These are called round ligaments, and stretching of these often causes discomfort, most commonly in the first trimester. Round ligament pain is usually perceived to be on both sides but may be worse on one side. However, severe one-sided pain in early pregnancy may be an indication of an ectopic pregnancy (pregnancy outside the uterus) and should be reported to your physician. The other most common discomfort of the first trimester is the nausea and vomiting referred to as morning sickness. If the vomiting becomes severe, the medical term applied is hyperemesis gravidarum. The cause of hyperemesis is still unknown, and it can be disabling in the most severe cases. However, the majority of women are able to tolerate this malaise without medical intervention, and most find that the nausea resolves in the early second trimester. Some women find that eating small meals of a diet high in starch helps to relieve the symptoms of hyperemesis.

The second and early third trimesters are considered to be the most comfortable times of pregnancy. By this time, the ligament stretching and nausea of the first trimester have resolved. At about seventeen weeks, the mother may experience the first sensations of fetal movement, referred to as quickening. Quickening is most often described as a fluttering sensation and has been mistaken for indigestion. However, as the fetus grows, the kicks become stronger, and the mother clearly recognizes them as purposeful movements.

In the last two months of pregnancy, the enlarging uterus begins to displace a number of abdominal organs, and symptoms are common. The diaphragm is elevated, resulting in shortness of breath. The uterus and the fetal head put pressure on the pelvic girdle and the lower back. Additionally, the ligaments that connect the pubic bones loosen in preparation for delivery, and sensations of pelvic laxity or instability with standing may result. The uterus also puts pressure on the veins that drain blood from the legs. As the blood flow slows, edema or swelling may result, and the veins become dilated. This may aggravate varicose veins and hemorrhoids. Swelling around the hands and wrists occasionally puts pressure on the nerves in these areas, resulting in painful tingling sensations. If these symptoms become severe, a wrist brace may be helpful. Finally, if the mother lies directly on her back, the large uterus puts significant pressure on the maternal blood vessels that lead to and from the heart. This slows blood return to the heart and causes a potentially serious drop in cardiac output. Therefore, in the last months of pregnancy, we recommend that women lie on their left or right side when in bed.

THE REPRODUCTIVE SYSTEM

The vulva, or the external genitalia of the mother, and the vagina are primarily affected by the greatly increased blood flow to this area. These structures change to a deeper and in some cases purplish hue, and vaginal secretions increase significantly throughout pregnancy. Together with the increased secretions of the cervix, the vaginal secretions are responsible for the well-known white discharge seen in pregnancy. The vaginal wall also undergoes changes, which prepare it for the enlargement necessary during childbirth. The lining of the vagina, or vaginal mucosa, increases in thickness. The amount of elastic and muscular tissue of the vaginal wall increases as well.

The uterine cervix also becomes much more vascular with pregnancy and changes in color to a bluish tint. The cervix softens, and the mucus-producing cells increase in size and number. These cells produce the "mucus plug." The function of this plug, or gelatinous collection of mucus, is unknown; it may protect from infection by preventing bacteria in the vagina from reaching the intrauterine environment. The mucus plug usually remains in place in the cervix until late in the pregnancy and is then passed as a preamble to labor. Similarly, the fibrous, elastic, and muscular components of the cervix increase significantly as pregnancy progresses, allowing the cervix to dilate during labor.

Of course, the most remarkable changes in the reproductive tract take place in the uterus. This unique female organ is capable of expanding up to one thousand times its nonpregnant volume to allow for the growth of the fetus. What begins as a thick-walled structure about the size of a small fist ends up as a large, hollow, thin-walled sac extending from deep in the pelvis to under the diaphragm. The uterus reaches rather predictable heights in the abdominal cavity depending on the weeks gestation of the pregnancy. By twelve weeks from the last menstrual period, the uterus can be felt at the pelvic brim, just above the pubic bone. By approximately twenty postmenstrual weeks, or halfway through the gestation, the top of the uterus reaches the navel, and thereafter it grows approximately one centimeter (about ½ inch) for every week until the last month of the pregnancy. The obstetrician uses a measuring tape to measure the uterus in the office on prenatal visits, providing a crude estimation of the gestational age of the pregnancy as well as week-to-week assurances that the fetus is continuing to grow.

THE BLOOD, VESSELS, AND HEART

Blood is composed of blood cells and a fluid component, plasma. During pregnancy, the red blood cells, which are responsible for carrying oxygen, increase by about 35 percent. The plasma volume increases even more, accounting for an overall increase in blood volume of nearly 50 percent. The greater increase in the plasma volume over the actual blood cells results in a drop in the proportion of red blood cells, or hematocrit. This "anemia of pregnancy" is a normal physiologic state resulting from normal changes in plasma and blood cell volume. The need for an increased number of iron-containing red cells is why iron supplementation is required during pregnancy. The increased blood volume is necessary to supply the mother, and indirectly the fetus, with adequate oxygen and nutrients. There is no direct connection between the blood systems of the mother and the fetus; instead, the transfer of nourishment takes place in the discoid, highly vascular fetal organ called the placenta. The maternal blood collects in large "lakes" at the base of the placenta. Here, the fetal blood vessels in the placenta come into indirect contact with the maternal blood, and vital compounds pass from the mother's blood through the placental cells and cells of the fetal blood vessel walls and finally into the fetal circulation.

The tendency of the blood to clot is enhanced with pregnancy. This is due to the increased production of some clotting factors as well as a decrease in the body's ability to lyse, or break down, clots that have already formed. Although the improved capacity to form clots is helpful in decreasing blood loss at the time of delivery, it is also responsible for a higher incidence of unwanted clots, especially in the veins of the legs.

Because of the increased demands of pregnancy, the maternal heart rate and function must increase. The amount of blood pumped per unit of time, or the cardiac output, progressively increases until it reaches one and one-half times the level of the nonpregnant state. The blood pressure of the normal pregnant woman drops during the middle part of pregnancy, the second trimester, and returns to a higher level toward the end of pregnancy. As mentioned earlier, a profound decrease in returning blood flow to the heart can be caused by the pressure of the pregnant uterus on the major blood vessels if the mother lies flat on her back for any extended period of time. This position is called the supine position, and it should be avoided during the second half of pregnancy.

The enlarged uterus and increased venous pressure in the legs leads to edema, or swelling caused by excess fluid retention. Most pregnant patients experience some swelling during pregnancy. This edema can be minimized by elevating the feet and legs and wearing support stockings. However, excessive edema, when associated with blood pressure elevation, brisk leg reflexes, and the spillage of unusual amounts of protein in the urine, is a sign of pre-eclampsia. Pre-eclampsia can lead to seizures and many other pregnancy complications.

THE RESPIRATORY SYSTEM

Many important changes occur in the respiratory system of the mother during pregnancy. These changes are responsible for the ability of the mother's blood to deliver more oxygen to her own tissues and to the utero-placental compartment. A slight shift in the pH (the acidity) of the mother's blood allows more oxygen to be released to the tissues. More oxygen is also available for diffusion across the placenta to the fetus. In turn, the carbon dioxide produced as a by-product of metabolism by both the fetal and maternal tissues is more readily picked up by her blood and delivered to the lungs for removal when she exhales.

During pregnancy, oxygen consumption increases by at least 15 percent. To meet this increased demand for oxygen, the maternal respiratory rate, as well as the total amount of air inspired during each breath, must increase.

Certain anatomical changes that affect respiration also occur with pregnancy. The rib cage flares at a greater angle, while the diaphragm is elevated to accommodate the growing uterus.

THE URINARY TRACT

Urination may be more frequent during pregnancy, and one reason for this is that the rate at which blood is filtered through the kidneys to produce urine increases by as much as 50 percent during pregnancy. This results in episodic loss of glucose and other nutrients in the urine, which would be an abnormal finding in an individual who was not pregnant. Because of this increase in filtration rate, the kidney is unable to reabsorb all of the nutrients that are lost in the urine, and the pregnant woman's urine may show small amounts of sugar, or glucose, when checked in the physician's office. On the other hand, significantly increased amounts of protein in the urine are unusual in pregnancy and may be a sign of kidney disease.

The ureters are tubes connecting the kidneys to the bladder. Urine from the kidneys flows through the two long ureters, which course down the posterior sides of the abdomen into the pelvis and to the bladder; the bladder then expels the urine through the urethra. During pregnancy, the enlarging uterus presses on the ureters, causing dilatation. Typically, the right ureter is dilated more than the left, primarily as a result of rotation of the uterus to the right. (The uterus is believed to rotate slightly to the right to accommodate the recto-sigmoid colon, which is located on the left side of the abdomen and pelvis.)

Urinary tract infections are a common complication of pregnancy. The infection may be without the usual symptoms of discomfort, and the mother is occasionally surprised to find that the infection exists. Therefore, frequent checks of the urine to detect this condition are important in prenatal care. Aside from a kidney infection, which may result in damage to the kidneys and could lead to a generalized infection of the bloodstream, urinary infections predispose the pregnant woman to premature labor and potentially premature birth.

THE DIGESTIVE SYSTEM

As a result of the enlarging uterus, the stomach and small intestines are elevated. The gastrointestinal tract is also slower to empty, which is believed to be caused by anatomical and hormonal changes. Because of the elevation of the stomach, the pressure within the stomach is higher than it is within the esophagus, and reflux of the acid stomach contents tends to cause heartburn.

The gallbladder can also be affected by pregnancy. It tends to enlarge and contains bile that is thicker than usual. Pregnancy is associated with an increased risk for the formation of gallstones, but in practice this is a rare complication.

THE SKIN AND MUSCULOSKELETAL SYSTEMS

Due mainly to hormonal effects, the skin of the palms tends to take on a reddish tint during pregnancy. Also, veins enlarge and become visible in the skin. Some of these veins are quite small and take on the appearance of tiny "spiders." The medical term for these small veins is spider angiomas. They form as a result of the increase in estrogen during pregnancy. Irregular light brownish patches may appear on the body, and especially on the face. This is called chloasma, which also appears in some women using birth control pills; it is primarily due to hormonal changes. After delivery, the patches become much lighter and are rarely unsightly.

Changes in the musculoskeletal system occur as the uterus enlarges. The mother becomes progressively swaybacked to compensate for the change in her center of gravity. Also, toward the end of pregnancy, the ligaments of the pelvic girdle begin to loosen in preparation for birth. As a result, symptoms such as pain and stretching in the back and pelvis are not unusual in the third trimester.

THE ENDOCRINE GLANDS

The major endocrine glands are the pituitary gland and the hypothalamus in the brain, the pancreas, the adrenal glands above the kidneys, and the thyroid and parathyroid glands in the neck. The ovaries in the woman and the testes in the man serve as endocrine and reproductive organs.

Growth of ovarian follicles stops during pregnancy. However, the ovary from which the follicle ovulated is important in the first eight weeks of pregnancy because it produces progesterone. Progesterone is necessary for the continuation of the pregnancy, and the major source of this hormone early in pregnancy is the corpus luteum of the ovary. The corpus luteum is a cystic structure that forms after ovulation and secretes the hormone progesterone until the placenta is sufficiently developed. Later in pregnancy, the placenta becomes the main source of progesterone.

The pituitary gland, at the base of the brain, enlarges somewhat during pregnancy. One of the substances produced by the pituitary gland is prolactin, which increases throughout pregnancy. After delivery, prolactin is important in maintaining lactation in the breast-feeding mother.

The thyroid gland may also enlarge during pregnancy. The gland produces increasing amounts of the thyroid hormones, but this is offset by an increase in proteins in the blood that bind hormones. Only the free hormones — those not bound to proteins in the blood — are active, so the overall effect of the thyroid gland remains unchanged with pregnancy.

The pancreas is responsible for producing two important hormones involved in the regulation of the blood sugar level: insulin and glucagon. Insulin promotes glucose (blood sugar) utilization and is secreted when the blood sugar rises. Insulin allows glucose to enter the tissues, where it can be utilized for metabolism; it also stimulates the production of proteins and the storage of lipids (fats). Glucagon, on the other hand, stimulates the production of blood glucose, not its storage. Therefore, in response to insulin the blood sugar level will fall, and in response to glucagon the blood sugar level will rise.

During pregnancy, more insulin is required to keep the blood sugar at its usual low level. If the pancreas has only a marginal ability to increase the secretion of insulin, the blood sugar may rise to unacceptably high values during pregnancy. This is why some women become borderline or even overtly diabetic during pregnancy. Their usual ability to secrete insulin from the pancreas in response to the increase in blood sugar following a meal is not sufficient to keep their blood sugar within normal range during pregnancy. Most patients who are not diabetic prior to pregnancy will require only a diet to control their glucose level during pregnancy. However, a few will require insulin for sugar control. This medication can be given at regular intervals during the day to optimize blood sugar control. After delivery, the insulin requirements again drop, and most women no longer require either a special diet or insulin to keep their glucose levels normal.

The parathyroid gland secretes parathormone, which along with vitamin D allows the body to reabsorb stored calcium from bone. In pregnancy, the mother's bones are protected from this bone breakdown by the action of another hormone, calcitonin. Calcitonin is secreted by the thyroid gland, and its level is known to increase during pregnancy and lactation.

The Physiology and Development of the Fetus

The story of the fetus actually begins long before conception, with the growth and development of the egg and sperm. The egg and sperm are special reproductive cells called gametes. They contain only half the number of chromosomes (gene-carrying structures) present in other cells, and thus when they unite form an embryo with genetic characteristics of both parents.

The eggs are present in a female long before she is born, about three weeks after conception. The eggs migrate to the ovaries, where they divide and mature through a complex process. A woman's ovaries contain about 2 million ova at the time of her birth. Only a small number of these are destined to become mature eggs. The rest degenerate at a rapid rate, leaving 500,000 present in the ovaries at the time of puberty. Of this half-million ova, about 500 will eventually ovulate during the reproductive life of a normal woman.

The primitive germ cells that give rise to spermatozoa in the father are also present in early embryonic life. They migrate to the testes during the fifth week after conception and there undergo division and maturation to give rise to mature sperm that are capable of fertilization. In the average ejaculate, or discharge of sperm-containing fluid, 140 million to 350 million sperm are present; but only a relatively small number of these will ever reach the fallopian tube to fertilize the mature egg. If a sperm is present to fertilize the egg at the optimal time after ovulation (within fifteen hours), and if the sperm successfully penetrates, the genetic material of the egg and sperm combines to form a zygote, which undergoes rapid cell division.

THE EMBRYO

Fertilization takes place in a special part of the fallopian tube called the ampulla. As the zygote divides, it is carried down the fallopian tube toward the uterus. There it burrows in, or implants, on the sixth day after conception and is nourished by the prepared uterine lining of pregnancy.

From fertilization through the first eight weeks of life, the conceptus is properly referred to as an embryo. During the embryonic period, all major organ systems form. This fact makes the embryo especially vulnerable to drugs or other teratogens that would cause little or no harm if encountered after the embryonic period.

The cells of the conceptus can be categorized as those destined to become the fetus itself and those destined to mature into the placenta and fetal membranes. These latter structures will be discussed in the next section. The embryo proper begins as a flat disk, which upon cell division curves into the body stalk. The embryo develops its bodily characteristics from the head downward in a way that is similar in all vertebrates. However, by the seventh week after fertilization, the embryo can be identified as distinctly human.

THE FETUS

From eight weeks postconception (ten weeks after the first day of the last menstrual period) until birth, the baby is known as a fetus. The fetal period is characterized by the growth and maturation of the body and organs that developed during the embryonic period.

The entire gestation lasts an average of 280 days, or 40 weeks. The 280 days can also be divided into 10 lunar months of 28 days each. The weight and size of the fetus increases rapidly as each lunar month progresses. At the close of the embryonic period (second lunar month) the weight is less than 10 grams (about ⅓ ounce), but by the fifth month, or 20 weeks, the fetus weighs at least 300 grams (10½ ounces). By seven months, or 28 weeks, the average fetus weighs just over 1000 grams (35 ounces), and by birth at 40 weeks, the fetus weighs over 3000 grams (6½ pounds).

THE FETAL CARDIAC AND RESPIRATORY SYSTEMS

The structure and function of the fetal cardiac and respiratory systems are dictated by the special environment of the uterus. Because there is no air in utero, the lungs are not expanded, and the fetus obtains all its oxygen from the mother's blood. The fetal circulatory system must bypass the unexpanded lungs and rely on oxygenated blood from the umbilical vein for metabolism. To do this, a number of special shunts (which close soon after birth) are present in the fetus. The carrier of oxygenated blood from the placenta to the fetus is the single umbilical vein. Blood flows through the umbilical vein into the liver, where the majority of oxygenated blood is directed to the heart through a special shunt called the ductus venosus. A connection between the left and right sides of the heart, called the foramen ovale, allows fresh blood to move rapidly across to the left side of the heart and out through the aorta to the carotid arteries to nourish the brain. The majority of blood that would pass through the lungs for oxygenation in the infant after birth is shunted through the ductus arteriosus and down to the remainder of the body in the unborn fetus. The blood returns via the two umbilical arteries to the placenta to pick up fresh oxygen and nutrients. All of these shunts are simply ways of rerouting precious oxygen and nutrients to the most important areas first and must close at birth for the adult type of circulation to be established. With the establishment of the adult pattern of circulation, all blood is routed through the lungs for oxygenation.

The Placenta and Fetal Membranes

The placenta is of fetal origin. Fetal cells called trophoblasts grow through the endometrial lining of the uterus and anchor themselves to the uterine wall. The divisions of the placenta are called cotyledons, and each is composed of a single main fetal blood vessel and its branches surrounded by trophoblastic cells. The maternal blood from the uterine arteries shoots out in spurts around each cotyledon. The needed nutrients then diffuse through the trophoblastic cells and fetal blood vessel walls. The many main and branching fetal blood vessels of the placenta then collect to form the one main vessel connecting it to the fetus, the umbilical vein. After circulation through the fetus, used (or deoxygenated) blood returns to the placenta through the umbilical arteries and circulates through the placenta again to pick up new oxygen.

The fetus grows in the amniotic sac. This sac is filled with amniotic fluid and is composed of a double membrane. The membrane closest to the fetus, or the inner membrane, is called the amnion. The outer membrane is called the chorion. The amnion and chorion form a barrier between the fetus and the outside world. They serve to hold in the amniotic fluid, which is necessary to the fetus, and to exclude bacteria from entering the cavity. Recently it has been demonstrated that the membranes may also be responsible for producing some important substances during pregnancy and probably allow chemical signals to pass between the fetus and mother. The fetal membranes usually remain intact until full term, when they may rupture either just before labor begins or during labor itself. If the membranes rupture early in gestation, many problems may be encountered, and any suspected leakage should be reported to your obstetrician.

After delivery of the infant, a cleavage line is created between the placenta and uterine lining. Within thirty minutes following birth, the placenta separates on its own and can be delivered by applying gentle traction.

In this chapter we have reviewed some of the structural and functional changes that take place in the mother's body during pregnancy. We have also reviewed the development of the embryo and fetus, and introduced you to the special organ of pregnancy, the placenta. The physiology of the mother, the fetus, and the placenta are closely interrelated, and must complement each other to ensure that a healthy new baby enters the world.

[PART III]

Establishing a Healthy Pregnancy Life-style

[7]

Nutrition:
Eating for One or Two
Kimberly K. Leslie, M.D.

There is no question that nutrition plays an important role in the health of a mother and her developing baby. And common sense tells us that adequate nutrition is desirable before the onset of pregnancy. The most important time to have an optimal environment for the developing baby is during the critical first eight weeks, when organ development occurs.

In the United States, overt malnutrition is uncommon. However, to assure an ideal nutritional state for pregnancy, we must consider excesses as well as deficiencies. This necessitates an adequate knowledge of which foods and what quantities are important for the developing fetus.

Nutrition has long been underrepresented in the medical school curriculum. Very few hours are devoted to this topic. That does not mean, however, that there is not a large body of information concerning good nutrition in pregnancy. To the contrary, a great deal is known, and an overview of this information is presented in this chapter.

PROPER NUTRITION is an important component of preparing for your pregnancy. We have become increasingly aware of the need for a well-balanced diet to maintain optimal health and conditioning. This concept is doubly significant during pregnancy, because it affects the fetus as well as the mother. Establishing healthful lifelong eating habits prior to conception will allow you to enter pregnancy in an optimal nutritional state and will provide you with adequate nutritional reserves for pregnancy.

Nutrition, the Science of Food

Nutrition is the science of food and the components of food that relate to health. There are some fifty known nutrients that are essential for proper body functioning. The nutrients are divided into six main categories: protein, carbohydrate, fat, minerals, vitamins, and water. Protein, carbohydrate, and fat are the only nutrients that provide calories for energy expenditure. Protein and carbohydrate each provide about 4 calories per gram, while fat provides about twice as many calories, or 9 per gram. Minerals and vitamins do not provide calories but are necessary for certain metabolic processes. Many enzymes that are important for body functions require specific minerals and vitamins for their activity. Also, minerals function as vital parts of body tissues, such as iron in hemoglobin and calcium in teeth and bones.

We know that the number of calories consumed during the day is important, but it is also important that the diet contain all of the vitamins and minerals required for metabolic activity. Since no single food provides all of the known nutrients, you should be sure to consume a varied diet. Also, you should not consume more calories than are required to reach and maintain a desirable body weight. The number of calories you need to maintain normal body weight depends upon your level of physical activity, and the easiest way to lose weight is to increase physical output while keeping the diet constant in caloric value.

In the last few decades, it has become increasingly clear that the quality of a person's diet can affect his or her health. Even though malnutrition per se is not rampant in the United States, if we describe or define malnutrition as any dietary habit that leads to poor health, it is common in all sectors of our society. High fat intake is related to atherosclerosis, which is manifested by coronary heart disease and cerebral and renal blood vessel disease. Essential hypertension (elevated blood pressure) certainly is aggravated by a diet with high sodium content. Also, the lack of fiber in our modern diets has been linked to the increase in colon cancer, irritable bowel syndrome, and diverticulitis seen in our society within the last hundred years.

It has been demonstrated in several studies that carefully controlled diets can decrease total serum cholesterol levels by more than 17 percent, significantly decreasing the risks of coronary artery disease in patients with high blood cholesterol. However, cholesterol restriction diets are less likely to reduce the serum cholesterol value of people who already have normal levels. Several types of cholesterol are present in the blood. The two main types are low-density lipoproteins (LDL) and high-density lipoproteins (HDL). Low-density lipoproteins are present in the highest concentration and place the patient at risk for atherosclerosis. HDL, on the other hand, is considered to be a "protective" form of cholesterol that, when present in high amounts, counteracts the dangers of LDL. Therefore, having a high HDL value and a low LDL value would be the most beneficial cholesterol composition. Dietary restriction of cholesterol can decrease the LDL level, while the HDL level remains constant.

The following are the primary aims in dietary management of high total serum cholesterol, and they are useful for anyone interested in healthful nutritional habits:

- Obtain a desirable overall body weight. This may entail some weight loss, which should be attained through moderately decreasing caloric intake while increasing physical activity.

- Lower the intake of saturated fat. Saturated fat tends to maintain high levels of LDL, while polyunsaturated fats lower LDL. The principal sources of saturated fat in the diet are meats and dairy products. Substitute fish and poultry for beef products, and use dairy products with lower fat content, such as skim milk, low-fat cottage cheese, sherbets, and so forth.
- Lower the dietary intake of cholesterol. The intake in an average diet is between 600 milligrams and 800 milligrams per day. This can be cut in half by limiting the use of egg yolks to two or three per week, while lessening consumption of organ meats, such as liver, and making other substitutions.
- Increase the intake of polyunsaturated fats. Polyunsaturated fats are found primarily in corn, soya, safflower, and cottonseed oils. Many margarines, cooking oils, and shortenings are made exclusively with polyunsaturated fats, and these should be the ones you choose.

By following these guidelines, it will be possible to decrease the amount of fat in your diet to about 35 percent of daily calories and to increase the ratio of polyunsaturated to saturated fat to about 1 to 1.

A type of malnutrition that we have not mentioned yet but is extremely prevalent in our society is obesity. An obese person has habitually taken in more calories than are necessary for body function and for energy expenditure. These extra calories have been stored as fat. Men or women whose weights are 20 percent or greater above their ideal body weight are at risk for cardiovascular and pulmonary diseases, diabetes, gallstones, and many orthopedic problems. A good therapeutic diet for obesity should provide all of the necessary nutrients in sufficient amounts but be restricted in calories. It has been shown that approximately one pound of fat represents the equivalent of 3500 calories. Thus a daily decrease in calories of approximately 500 will lead to an average weekly weight loss of one pound. It should be remembered that a decrease in caloric intake of 200 calories per day associated with an increase in energy expenditure of 300 calories per day would accomplish the same effect as a decrease of 500 calories per day in the diet alone. A weight loss of between one to two pounds per week is the best way to lose weight over the long term. It is not recommended that a man consume fewer than 1500 calories per day, nor a woman fewer than 1000 calories per day.

Even patients on weight-reduction diets should remember to have a balanced diet. A balanced diet is composed of the following: 12 percent to 14 percent of the calories should come from protein, 35 to 40 percent of the calories from fat, and the rest should be provided by carbohydrates. Probably the best way to maintain a diet such as this is to eat well-balanced meals but in smaller proportions, and to decrease the intake of sweets. Many formula diets are on the market. Their chief advantage is that they are easy to use, and the best ones provide a well-balanced nutritional package. They are especially useful in the beginning of a weight-control program, or to substitute for one meal a day. However, fad diets that rely on eating only certain foods or large quantities of one or two food groups are to be avoided.

A lack of fiber in the American diet has been proposed to be a cause of the recent increase in colon cancer, appendicitis, irritable bowel syndrome, and diverticular disease. Fiber is the part of plant material which is not easily digested. Fiber includes carbohydrate compounds such as cellulose and pectin. Fiber increases fecal bulk and produces more frequent and softer stools. A high-fiber diet can be helpful in treating constipation, a common complaint during pregnancy, with none of the adverse effects of laxatives. A high-fiber diet has also been beneficial in treating patients with hemorrhoids, another ailment typically associated with pregnancy. Evidence has been mounting that a diet high in soluble fiber, such as pectin, can decrease serum cholesterol. There has been an association between populations whose mean serum cholesterols are low (and who have a low incidence of coronary artery disease) and whose diets are high in fiber. Although the mechanism isn't known, we theorize that high-fiber diets may increase the body's excretion of cholesterol breakdown products, or decrease the absorption of cholesterol from the intestine.

Leading Up to Pregnancy

Poor nutrition, particularly when associated with dramatic weight loss, can decrease a woman's ability to ovulate, or produce an egg, on a regular basis. It can also affect the birth weight of her baby. Your prepregnancy nutritional status is a major predictor of your baby's birth weight. Weight compared to height is a measure physicians will often use to assess the status of a woman's current nutritional state, and normal maternal weight for height before pregnancy correlates well with normally grown infants at birth.

We believe that all babies are genetically "programmed" to reach a certain birth weight, which depends upon the size characteristics inherited from their parents. Some infants fail to reach their potential birth weight because they lack adequate food stores for growth. This leads to the clinical syndrome called intrauterine growth retardation. Babies who are growth retarded are at risk for problems during gestation, as well as in the nursery postnatally. Prenatally, growth-retarded fetuses are at a greater risk than their well-grown peers for premature birth, heart rate patterns suggestive of distress, and even death. After birth, these babies must be watched closely in the nursery and they may manifest dangerously low blood levels of glucose (sugar) and calcium. One of the most common causes of intrauterine growth retardation is the lack of adequate calories in the diet of the mother during pregnancy. A diet that deviates significantly from the recommended norms may put the pregnancy in jeopardy.

It is important to understand, however, that providing caloric supplementation to women who already have adequate diets does not improve pregnancy outcome. Overeating on the premise that the pregnancy will be benefited results only in maternal obesity and in a greater potential for the development of gestational diabetes in patients who are predisposed.

In the moderately active, healthy woman, a nutritionally balanced and complete diet can be achieved by eating from all major food groups to attain a caloric intake of approximately 2100 calories per day. We recommend that women planning to get pregnant start taking specially formulated prenatal multivitamin-multimineral tablets a few months before pregnancy to ensure that their vitamin and mineral stores are sufficient.

Most people understand that they should eat from different food groups, they understand that they should eat a variety of foods, and they understand that they should not eat sweets. However, understanding and doing are two different things. How people can be motivated to do what they know is healthful remains a major problem in dietary control. Here are a few suggestions for improving your eating habits:

- Keep your caloric intake relatively constant from day to day (about 2100 calories per day for an average woman).
- Don't snack between meals, and especially prior to bedtime, which puts you at the greatest risk for obesity.
- Choose a variety of nutritious foods, and don't limit

your choices to several well-liked foods, because the nutritional value in these foodstuffs may leave you short of various nutrients.

· Limit sweets, because sweets supply calories but tend to be relatively low in other types of nutrients; these calories could be better spent if confined to more nutritionally sound foods.

Resisting sweets and other foods with high calorie counts to maintain your most healthy weight requires constant vigilance. Unfortunately, many young women have acquired dangerous habits in an attempt to keep that perfect figure. Anorexia nervosa and bulimia are two examples of destructive behaviors that can be life-threatening. If you suspect that you have an obsession with thinness, and are constantly dieting despite the advice of others, or rely on induced vomiting to maintain your weight, we urge you to seek professional help!

What is your ideal body weight? Actually, many tables and graphs depict ideal body weight, but perhaps the easiest and most practical system of determining it can be computed with simple addition. To begin, assume that a five-foot-tall woman should weigh 100 pounds, and add 5 pounds for each additional inch of height. Of course, this is just a guideline or rule of thumb. An actual determination of ideal body weight must take into account factors like stature, frame, and physical condition.

A good diet can be instituted with the help of your nutritionist or local chapter of Weight Watchers. In general, however, we recommend a varied and balanced diet that relies on eating healthful foods from all food groups, but in lesser quantities. Most women will lose weight slowly but steadily while consuming 1000 to 1500 calories per day. A balanced exercise program such as that described in the next chapter, combining muscle strengthening, aerobics, and specific muscle group toning, can be of enormous help in reducing fat and increasing muscle while dieting.

It is important for a woman to be at or near her ideal weight *prior to* pregnancy. If her body weight is significantly under the ideal, she will have to gain proportionately more weight during pregnancy to prevent her baby from potentially becoming growth retarded. To state it another way, a woman who enters pregnancy significantly underweight (that is, less than 90 percent of her ideal body weight) definitely has to gain more weight during her pregnancy in order to keep the pregnancy at low risk. This is difficult for many underweight people to do, especially in the first or second trimester. Women who are significantly over their ideal body weight going into pregnancy (between 20 percent and 30 percent above their ideal body weight for their frame size and height) will usually gain less weight during pregnancy. However, these women may have complications during pregnancy. It is much more difficult to perform surgery if necessary on patients who are obese, and they are at greater risk in the postsurgical period. Also, as mentioned earlier, patients who have a genetic predisposition to diabetes will manifest it more readily if they are obese during pregnancy.

We do not recommend weight reduction during pregnancy itself, because the fetus is sensitive to both low maternal blood glucose levels and high maternal ketone levels. Ketones are breakdown products from fat, and if a patient is continually breaking down fat and not supplying enough glucose, the fetus can suffer metabolic disorders.

Nutrition During Pregnancy

The study of nutrition, like medicine as a whole, is a combination of art and science. Over the last several decades, professionals in the field of nutrition have undergone considerable evolution in their thinking regarding the proper nutritional recommendations for pregnancy. It can be stated with certainty that these recommendations are bound to change as new information comes to light. However, hard scientific data about nutrition in pregnancy depends upon well-controlled studies, which are often impossible to perform with humans for ethical reasons.

The milestone studies concerning maternal nutrition demonstrate the evolution in the field of nutrition quite well and are worth reviewing briefly. In 1943, B. S. Burke and others, in a study of women in Boston, were able to show a high correlation between favorable pregnancy outcomes and adequate maternal nutrition. Based on this study, prospective mothers were encouraged to gain increasing amounts of weight during pregnancy. However, subsequent studies such as that published in 1959 by Thomson in Aberdeen refuted the role of increased nutritional supplementation on improving the quality of pregnancy. This investigation initiated a shift to the viewpoint that the caloric intake of the mother did not need to increase to provide for the nutritional needs of the fetus. However, in the last two decades, it has been shown that maternal weight gain during pregnancy is a major factor influencing birth weight and fetal well-being. The public as a whole and professionals in the field have developed a renewed belief that adequate nutrition is extremely important for health.

The Food and Nutrition Board of the National Research Council has recommended an increase of 300 calories per day for the pregnant woman. That is, the average woman should increase her daily intake from 2100 calories to 2400 calories. Tables 7-1 and 7-2 summarize the currently recommended nutritional needs of the pregnant woman and the foods that contain these nutrients. Women in their teens have higher basic requirements of some nutrients. This is because teenagers are still growing. They have to supply

TABLE 7-1
DAILY NUTRITIONAL NEEDS OF PREGNANT WOMEN

Nutrient	Nonpregnant	In Pregnancy	Need for Increase	Food Sources
Calories	2100	2400	Protein-sparing energy needs	Carbohydrates (45–55%) Fats (35–40%) Protein (12–14%)
Protein	44 gm	74–100 gm	Fetal growth Placenta growth and development Maternal tissues, uterus, breast Increased maternal circulation Maternal stores for delivery and lactation	Meat Fish Poultry Cheese Eggs Legumes
Calcium	800 mg*	1200 mg†	Fetal skeleton and tooth formation	Milk Cheese Egg yolk Whole grains Leafy green vegetables

TABLE 7-1 (*continued*)
DAILY NUTRITIONAL NEEDS OF PREGNANT WOMEN

Nutrient	Nonpregnant	In Pregnancy	Need for Increase	Food Sources
Phosphorus	800 mg*	1200 mg†	Fetal skeleton and tooth formation Maternal phosphorus metabolism	Milk Cheese Lean meats
Iron	18 mg	18 mg, plus 30–60 mg supplementation	Maintain hemoglobin level Furnish iron for fetal development	Pork liver and kidney Beef liver Oysters Clams Prune juice Raisins Cooked dried beans Dried apricots Dried prunes
Iodine	150 µg	175 µg	Increased basal metabolic rate Increased thyroxine (thyroid hormone) production	Iodized salt

Magnesium	300 mg	450 mg	Coenzyme in energy and protein metabolism	Leafy green vegetables Dates, figs Whole grains
Zinc	15 mg	20 mg	Role in metabolism helps to maintain acid/base balance in tissues Growth Wound healing	Meat Liver Eggs Seafood Oysters
Vitamin A	800 µg (4000 IU)	1000 µg (5000 IU)	Essential for cell development, tooth bud formation, healthy skin Vision (light/dark adaptation)	Butter Egg yolk Fortified margarine Kidney Liver Whole milk Cream
Vitamin D	5–10 µg (200–400 IU)	15 µg (400–600 IU)	Absorption of calcium and phosphorus for growth and formation of bones and teeth	Butter Egg yolk Fish oils Liver Fortified milk

TABLE 7-1 (*continued*)
DAILY NUTRITIONAL NEEDS OF PREGNANT WOMEN

Nutrient	Nonpregnant	In Pregnancy	Need for Increase	Food Sources
Vitamin E	8 mg	10 mg	Tissue growth Cell wall integrity	Vegetable oils Leafy green vegetables Wheat germ Nuts Whole grains
Vitamin C	60 mg	80 mg	Tissue formation Increase iron absorption	Citrus fruits Berries Tomatoes Broccoli Potatoes

Folic acid	400 μg	800 μg	Normal cell division
			Increased metabolic demand
			Prevention of megaloblastic
			  anemia in high-risk patients
			Increased heme production for
			  hemoglobin
				Liver
				Leafy green vegetables
				Wheat germ

Niacin	13 mg	15 mg	Coenzyme in energy metabolism Coenzyme in protein metabolism	Meat Peanuts Fish Eggs Legumes Enriched grains
Riboflavin	1.2 mg	1.5 mg	Metabolism of amino acids and carbohydrates	Heart Kidney Liver Milk Enriched grains

* Adolescents need 1200 mg.
† Adolescents need 1600 mg.
gm = gram   mg = milligram   µg = microgram   IU = international unit

TABLE 7-2
SUGGESTED MEAL PATTERN FOR PREGNANCY

Food Group	Recommended Daily Intake	Comments
Milk (whole or skim, or butter-milk, or evaporated), yogurt, cheese, cottage cheese	Four servings Count as one serving: 1 cup milk ¾ cup yogurt 1½ oz. hard cheese ½ cup cottage cheese	
Meat, fish, poultry, eggs; dry peas, beans, lentils; nuts, peanut butter	Two or more servings Count as one serving: 4 oz. meat, fish, poultry 1 egg 1 cup cooked dried beans 3 tablespoons peanut butter	Liver at least once per week
Fruit	Two or more servings Count as one serving: 1 small fruit ½ cup juice 1 cup fruit pieces	One serving should be a citrus fruit or another source of ascorbic acid

TABLE 7-2 (*continued*)
SUGGESTED MEAL PATTERN FOR PREGNANCY

Food Group	Recommended Daily Intake	Comments
Vegetables	Two or more servings Count as one serving: ½ cup cooked vegetables 1 cup raw vegetables	Include ½ cup dark green leafy or deep yellow vegetables, ½ cup to 1 cup other vegetables
Breads and cereals	Four or more servings Count as one serving: 1 slice bread ½ cup cooked noodles, spaghetti, rice, macaroni ½ cup cooked cereal ⅔-1 cup dry cereal flakes 5-6 saltines	Include whole-grain or enriched breads, crackers, macaroni, spaghetti, noodles, rice, grits, tortillas, cornmeal, and cooked or ready-to-eat cereal

enough calories and minerals and vitamins not only for their own metabolic processes, but also for growth. This is doubly true for pregnant teens, who are now trying to supply their own growth, plus the growth of the fetus, plus their basic metabolic requirements. They are definitely at risk for inadequate nutrition during pregnancy.

WEIGHT GAIN

As alluded to earlier, the appropriate amount of weight to gain in pregnancy is again becoming a controversial issue among health professionals. It is known that at least twenty pounds must be gained by the mother during pregnancy to account for the weight of the average baby, placenta, increased fluid and blood volumes, and larger size of the uterus and breasts. Prior to 1986, the American College of Obstetricians and Gynecologists recommended that the average weight gain during pregnancy be twenty-two to twenty-seven pounds. However, recent data generated by the National Center for Health Statistics suggests that the optimal weight gain is more likely to be between twenty-six and thirty-five pounds. It has also been shown that women who are underweight prior to pregnancy tend to gain more weight, while obese women gain less.

The total amount of weight gained is important, but the rate at which it is gained is equally so. Excessively rapid weight gain, for example, can put you at risk for some of the complications mentioned earlier, or it can make you want to cut back on calories in the later stages of pregnancy, when the fetus is growing most quickly. For the first eight weeks of pregnancy, virtually no weight is gained. During the rest of the first trimester, weight increases slowly, normally about two to three pounds in all. The rate of gain increases thereafter, averaging about a pound every nine days, then leveling off just after week forty. You and your physician will work out a weight-gain plan for you, based on your current nutritional state.

IRON AND FOLIC ACID

Two nutrients deserve special attention during pregnancy: iron and folic acid. During the second half of pregnancy, a total of between 600 and 900 milligrams of iron is required to support the additional red blood cells needed by the mother as well as to allow development of the fetal blood supply. The iron must come from dietary intake or maternal stores. Because menstruation may result in the depletion of iron stores in the average woman, many women do not begin pregnancy with enough stores to supply themselves and their fetuses adequately. It is for this reason that iron supplements are often recommended during pregnancy. The addition of 30 to 60 milligrams of iron per day ensures that this nutrient will be available in quantities sufficient to meet the increased needs of pregnancy.

Folic acid is a nutrient that is rarely in short supply in the average U.S. diet. Although folic acid is most abundant in fresh leafy vegetables, even processed foods generally contain enough folic acid to maintain health in the pregnant state. However, because of its absolute necessity for the proper growth of tissues and because of some studies linking its deficiency to poor outcomes (including anything from neural tube defects to fetal death in utero), folic acid is also provided in supplement form to many pregnant women.

EXERCISE AND NUTRITION

Special consideration regarding nutritional requirements must be given to the woman who exercises regularly. The chapter on exercise before and during pregnancy encourages the establishment of a regular exercise program that can be continued in a modified form throughout pregnancy. Of course, exercise, especially aerobic exercise, requires increased caloric intake. Depending on the frequency and intensity of your exercise program, your daily intake of calories should increase to between 2500 and 3500 calories as needed to maintain a desirable rate of weight gain. Daily protein intake from the diet needs to increase by an average of 20 grams over and above the increase required by pregnancy alone, while calcium intake should increase by approximately 200 milligrams. Some increase in iron supplementation is usually recommended as well.

Too Much of a Good Thing

Some individuals take vitamin supplements in large quantities in the nonpregnant state. This is unnecessary and possibly dangerous.

It is important to be aware of the potential danger of oversupplementing some common vitamins. Several vitamins and minerals, when ingested in megadoses, can result in damaging effects on the fetus. Specifically, high doses of vitamins A, B_6, C, and D, and of iodine have been implicated as potential causes of birth defects.

A woman taking megadoses of vitamins should stop immediately; then she should wait several months before becoming pregnant. There are many properly formulated prenatal vitamin preparations. They contain vitamins, iron, and folate. Those containing higher levels of folate are by prescription only. We recommend using these time-tested preparations in order to avoid receiving excessive doses of any vitamin.

The most important concept presented here is the need for "good old common sense." Eating a balanced diet that provides calories from foods with good nutritional value is one of the most important contributions any woman can make to her pregnancy. Obviously, avoiding too many sweets and other fattening foods is included in this mandate. But, fortunately, once ideal body weight is achieved, maintaining good habits becomes routine and even enjoyable. The only real "work" involved with diet and nutrition is decreasing or increasing weight to reach ideal body weight. A balance of good nutrition, exercise, and rest can make you feel better day to day. You will enjoy your pregnancy more if you take good care of yourself.

Good luck and bon appetit!

[8]

Exercise: Become Fit Before You Get Pregnant
Mona M. Shangold, M.D.

Today, we all know the theoretical advantages of keeping ourselves in good physical condition through proper nutrition and regular exercise programs. A physically strong body affords major advantages for the woman who is planning to become pregnant. There is evidence to suggest that individuals who are physically fit tolerate pregnancy and delivery better. Although extremes of exercise may not be beneficial to the pregnancy, we recommend regular exercise programs and/or sports for women planning pregnancy.

In the past, the pregnant mother was believed to be in a "delicate state," and restriction of activities and even bed rest were commonly recommended for mothers during pregnancy. Following delivery, the mother having a first baby stayed in the hospital seven days, and the mother having subsequent children often stayed five days. Today, the mother is encouraged to exercise before and during pregnancy, and after delivery she is instructed to ambulate as quickly as possible. This speeds her recovery and helps to prepare her for an earlier discharge. The average hospital stay following an uncomplicated vaginal birth is now between two and three days. This change to a philosophy supporting more physical activity during pregnancy and less time in the hospital is a trend that is popular with both health professionals and patients. In this chapter, the importance of a regular exercise program for physical fitness is emphasized and exercise guidelines for pregnancy are given.

THE KEY TO FITNESS during pregnancy is fitness before pregnancy. It is unfortunate that many women become interested in exercise for the first time while pregnant. They would be much wiser to strive for fitness *before* pregnancy. Pregnancy itself is hard work, and it is much easier to perform this hard work if you are already physically fit. A pregnant body does a lot of work in merely nourishing a baby. Any activity done while carrying the extra weight of pregnancy presents an even greater work load than would be presented in the nonpregnant state. Women who are poorly conditioned when they become pregnant are often unable to carry on routine activities without considerable fatigue. You should aim to become fit before you become pregnant and to maintain a level of fitness during pregnancy.

Consider your pregnancy to be a training supplement rather than an inconvenience. Pregnancy is analogous to running a marathon. You wouldn't enter such an athletic event without appropriate training. Similarly, you should prepare your body for pregnancy with a cardiovascular conditioning program. Having a strong heart muscle will enable you to do the work of pregnancy with much less effort.

If you haven't exercised previously, start now. Ideally, you should begin training at least one year before becoming pregnant; at a minimum, you should begin three months ahead of time. The major reason for beginning a training program at least three months prior to pregnancy is to allow your body time to undergo the changes that occur with regular exercise before it is subjected to the demands of pregnancy. If you haven't developed a regular exercise program by the time you read this book and are planning a pregnancy more than three months from now, you should certainly begin exercising as soon as possible.

Why Exercise?

Most women who become interested in exercise during pregnancy do so for one of two reasons. Some think that a healthful life-style, including exercise, will benefit the baby; others hope to avoid getting fat, a common problem for many pregnant women. Although it has not been proven that exercise will improve the outcome of your pregnancy, it is probable that women who exercise regularly *feel* better than women who do not. Adequate exercise, combined with a sensible diet, is the most effective way of avoiding the accumulation of fat in the first place, but pregnancy is not a good time to try to lose fat. Losing fat requires burning more calories than you take in, that is, having a calorie deficit. This is not desirable during pregnancy because it reduces the calories and nutrients available to feed the growing fetus. This could harm the baby's growth, regardless of whether the deficit is created by dieting or by exercise. The time to lose fat is before pregnancy. Most nonpregnant women try to eliminate fat by dieting alone. This is usually counterproductive since dieting slows down the metabolic rate, thus slowing down the rate at which the body uses up calories. Exercise, on the other hand, accelerates the metabolic rate, making it easier to get rid of fat. Exercise also promotes formation of muscle tissue. Since muscle tissue is active, while fat tissue is inert, muscle uses more energy than fat. A muscular person will burn more calories than a fat person of the same weight during any activity or while at rest.

Aerobic and Resistance Exercise

Two types of exercise are important for all women: aerobic and resistance. Aerobic exercise refers to activities that are done continuously, leading to sustained elevation of heart rate. This type of exercise includes sports like swimming and cross-country skiing, as well as activities such as brisk walking, jogging, stationary bicycling, and aerobic dancing. Aerobic exercise strengthens the heart muscle and also burns a lot of calories. Tennis is not aerobic exercise for most of us because we are not able to keep the ball going back and forth long enough to keep us moving continuously. (Every time we stop to pick up the balls, most of us do so at a slow pace, allowing our heart rates to slow down. This interferes with the cardiovascular benefit.) Sports like volleyball also involve much starting and stopping, thereby preventing the sustained elevation of heart rate needed for heart benefit. Resistance exercise refers to strength training, that is, contracting your muscles against resistance, as is done when you lift weights. Resistance training strengthens muscles and bones and leads to a faster metabolic rate because it develops more muscle tissue. Thus, all women should be involved in both aerobic exercise and resistance training.

CARDIOVASCULAR FITNESS

To attain and maintain cardiovascular fitness, your aerobic exercise before pregnancy should include thirty minutes of continuous exertion at a level vigorous enough to keep your heart rate at 100 or more beats per minute, and you should repeat such exercise two or three times each week, on alternate days. This is the minimum amount of exercise necessary to strengthen your heart muscle and keep it strong. More intense exercise will lead to even greater fitness, but it will also increase your chance of being injured. Longer durations of aerobic exercise (more than thirty minutes per session) and greater frequency of exercise (more often than two or three times a week) will lead to slight improvement in fitness and much improvement in caloric expenditure. This is an excellent way to lose weight or keep fat off.

If you are beginning an aerobic exercise program following a previously sedentary life-style, plan to begin at a slow pace. Choose the activity that suits you best, based on what you enjoy and what is available to you. If you have to drive two hours to reach a swimming pool, it is unlikely you will be able to incorporate swimming into your regular routine; or if you live at a very cold location where the ground is covered by snow for several months of the year, an outdoor running program will probably be short-lived.

Now, suppose your chosen sport is running. How should you proceed? You might begin your program by running for a few minutes, at a pace that is comfortable enough to carry on a conversation, and then walking for a few minutes. Continue alternating for a total of about fifteen minutes in the first session. In the beginning, you may find that brisk walking is about as much as you can do. Do not be discouraged. You will gradually find that you can run longer and longer without tiring your leg muscles. If you find that you are gasping for breath, you are probably going too fast. Over the course of three to four weeks, you should gradually increase the amount of time you are running, to the point where you can run continuously for thirty minutes. It is better to err on the slow side and build up gradually than to overdo and be injured. An injury early will set you back and delay the progression of your program. Listen to your body. It may take a while to overcome years of a sedentary life-style, but you will soon be pleasantly surprised by your own improvement.

If you are in good health, you can probably begin this exercise program without consulting your physician. However, if you have any medical problems, you should certainly discuss any exercise plans with your physician before you begin. If you experience any symptoms during exercise, such as lightheadedness, dizziness, chest pain, or more shortness of breath than can be accounted for by the exercise itself, you should certainly consult your physician before you continue exercising.

MUSCULAR STRENGTH

Your resistance training program should also be practiced two or three times each week, preferably on alternate days. To strengthen each group of muscles, you should lift the heaviest weight you can lift ten times in succession. If you can lift a given weight more than ten times in succession, the weight is too light to strengthen your muscles significantly. If you cannot lift it ten times, the weight is too heavy for you. Practice a series of exercises intended to strengthen a number of different muscle groups, including biceps and triceps (front and back of the upper arms), deltoids (shoulders), pectorals (upper chest), upper and lower back muscles, quadriceps and hamstrings (front and back of the thighs), and abdominal muscles. As your pregnancy progresses, abdominal muscle exercises may be uncomfortable, and you may choose to avoid them after this time.

Because each of your muscle groups has a unique amount of inherent strength, the appropriate amount of resistance for each group is also unique. Therefore, you will not lift the same amount of weight in doing different exercises. The stronger a muscle group, the heavier the weight you should lift with it in order to maintain or increase its strength. Weaker muscle groups (such as the triceps) will not be able to lift as much weight as stronger ones (such as the quadriceps) and will require lighter weights. It is quite possible for a woman to require 20 pounds of weight in each of ten repetitions for some muscle groups and 170 pounds in each of ten repetitions for others.

Your weight training can be accomplished using either free weights or weight-training machines, such as home exercise or Nautilus equipment. Free weights are less expensive, but they are more time-consuming since you must stop and manually change the weights for each of the different muscle groups. To change the amount of weight while you exercise with machines, on the other hand, requires moving only one pin. However, weight machines require a great initial financial expenditure or access to a facility that has such equipment.

If you have never lifted weights before, you will probably benefit from visiting a health club that has a knowledgeable instructor for initial guidance. After you have learned the fundamentals and have determined the appropriate amount of weight for each of several muscle groups, you can probably continue safely on your own.

Some Precautions

Although it is helpful for pregnant women to exercise, certain precautions are appropriate because doctors don't know the upper limits of safe exercise for developing babies. The mother's physical fitness is certainly important, but it should not compromise the baby's well-being. Doctors don't know how intensely a woman can exercise before a significant amount of blood will be diverted from the uterus, and this might diminish the oxygen and nutrients that enable the fetus to grow and develop normally. During exercise, more blood flows to the exercising muscles, while less flows to other organs, such as the uterus. It is likely that more blood will be diverted away from the uterus at higher levels of intensity. So to be on the safe side, for example, a woman who is a competitive runner should probably avoid speed work during her pregnancy.

High temperatures in early pregnancy may lead to an increased risk of certain types of birth defects. Continuous (aerobic) exercise leads to an increase in muscle temperature, which may raise the temperature of the entire body. This is unlikely to happen before thirty minutes of exercise have been completed, although some women may have an increase in temperature shortly after thirty minutes have passed. At some point in early pregnancy, you should probably check your rectal temperature at the end of your customary exercise, no matter what the duration, to be sure that it does not exceed 101 degrees Fahrenheit. It should be necessary to do this only once; you can assume that your temperature will be about the same following a similar intensity and duration of exercise at any stage of pregnancy. If your temperature is too high, take some measures to keep cooler, such as exercising at a cooler time of day, wearing lighter clothing, or exercising for shorter duration. Be sure to consume enough fluids when you exercise, particularly since dehydration promotes a temperature rise. In general, it is probably sensible for pregnant women to limit their exercise sessions to thirty minutes.

Exercise Guidelines for Pregnancy

If you are planning to exercise aerobically during pregnancy, you should do so in the same activity you were involved in prior to pregnancy, and your aerobic exercise should be of no greater intensity than you were accustomed to before. Since you are exercising with added weight, and since your body is doing more work merely by being pregnant, you will need to slow down considerably compared to your prepregnancy pace. If you were not used to regular aerobic exercise before pregnancy, you should practice no aerobic exercise more vigorous than brisk walking.

Some women should not exercise aerobically during pregnancy. If you have any obstetrical complication, you should certainly discuss this with your doctor before engaging in an exercise program.

Even if you were not accustomed to exercising in any way before pregnancy, weight training is a good idea during pregnancy; you can follow the same progression you would if you weren't pregnant. You will strengthen your muscles and bones from such resistance exercise, and your stronger muscles will be less likely to cause low back pain and other muscular aches and pains common to pregnant women. The stronger muscles you develop will also make it easier for you to carry your baby around after birth. The only women who should not lift weights during pregnancy are those with heart disease or muscle injuries. Although calisthenics are acceptable, they will not make you fit or strong.

Nutrition is of concern for exercising pregnant women because they must provide enough calories for themselves, the pregnancy, and the exercise. Although more calories are needed, the exercising pregnant woman does not need much more of any specific nutrients than her sedentary pregnant friends, only a few vitamins that are required in proportion to energy expenditure. In any event, these vitamins (thiamine, niacin, riboflavin, and pantothenic acid) are provided adequately in a well-balanced diet, so there is no need to be concerned about them as long as the pregnant exerciser eats sufficient calories, as discussed in Chapter 6.

Although it is reasonable for most women to gain twenty-five to thirty-five pounds during pregnancy, doctors don't know if the same range is appropriate for pregnant exercisers. However, this goal is probably reasonable for exercisers too, particularly if you are gaining weight and growing at the appropriate rate.

Finally, it is obvious that you should avoid any activities that lead to a risk of abdominal trauma, such as downhill skiing or horseback riding, since this might endanger your baby. In summary, you should become fit before you become pregnant and should try to maintain a level of fitness throughout pregnancy. This will probably make you feel better during pregnancy and make it easier for you to get back in shape after the baby is born.

[9]

Medications and Environment
Kimberly K. Leslie, M.D.

Numerous studies have shown that normal women take an average of four prescription medications during the course of a pregnancy. This number does not include the many over-the-counter remedies that may be taken during gestation, often without much thought. Although most of these medications are probably safe during pregnancy, why take the chance? Because some may be harmful to the fetus, the following chapter is obviously important; it outlines medications known to be teratogenic (capable of producing congenital malformations).

We are also often asked about nonmedicinal agents such as caffeine, alcohol, and nicotine. It is clear that all three of these easily cross the placenta and enter the baby's circulation. And evidence grows daily that the use of so-called recreational drugs during pregnancy poses a serious threat to a baby's well-being. The guiding principle concerning any chemical or medication should be: Would you give this to your newborn baby?

There are similar potential hazards arising from extremes in the environment — for instance, very high temperatures causing hyperthermia, or exposures to certain chemicals. This chapter attempts to put this information into perspective so that you may proceed through pregnancy with a feeling of confidence instead of concern.

Exposure to some medications and environmental factors should be minimized during pregnancy. Actually, the list of agents that have been proven to cause fetal defects is surprisingly small. They are called teratogens, meaning capable of causing fetal malformations, and include infectious organisms, certain drugs, ionizing radiation, some maternal diseases, and hyperthermia. Teratology is a relatively new field of study, and there are many agents that have not been thoroughly tested and about which little scientific evidence is known. It should also be remembered that much of the data that is available is derived from studies on laboratory animals. Since many experiments would be difficult or unethical to perform in pregnant women, the animal model is indispensable; but it is not completely accurate. A sad example of this dilemma is the thalidomide disaster. This drug, a mild sedative, was tested and found to cause no damage in rats and mice, but it turned out to be highly teratogenic in humans. Conversely, some medications have been found to cause fetal defects in laboratory animals but not in humans. Therefore, until better experimental methods are available yielding more complete information, we must rely largely on common sense. It is wise to avoid known environmental hazards and medications or drugs not prescribed by your physician. Over-the-counter medications may indeed be safe, but you should consult your doctor before taking them if you think you could be pregnant. With few exceptions, all drugs are believed to cross the placenta and enter the fetal circulation.

In general, the timing of exposure to teratogenic agents

is the most important factor in evaluating the potential effects on pregnancy. During organ system formation (organogenesis), in the first trimester, the fetus is most vulnerable to damage. In most cases, exposure later in gestation leads to less severe consequences. It is also known that even dangerous environmental factors, when encountered very early in pregnancy (the first two weeks after conception), rarely lead to the birth of a defective infant. The consequences of these early exposures represent the "all-or-none" phenomenon: the conceptus dies, or it develops normally. The relative safety of the first two post-conceptual weeks centers around the ability of the undamaged cells to grow and take over the function of the cells that were injured or died as a result of the insult. However, following this relatively safe period, the embryo enters its most vulnerable developmental stage, lasting until the end of the embryonic period, or about eight weeks after conception. Even after organogenesis, tissue growth and development continue. Significant exposures after this time primarily affect organs like the brain, which undergo active growth and development after the embryonic stage.

With this introduction in mind, let's review the list of known teratogens.

Infectious Agents

The viruses herpes, varicella (chickenpox), rubella (three-day measles), and cytomegalovirus are known or suspected to be teratogenic. In general, these agents can cause profound developmental defects if contracted in utero; however, the attack rate is highly variable. Many fetuses may be unaffected, while others will be significantly damaged. Except for herpes, in which only rare cases have been reported, the viruses easily cross the placenta from mother to child. If the mother becomes infected during the embryonic period, the results to a fetus that also contracts

TABLE 9-1
KNOWN AND SUSPECTED HUMAN TERATOGENS

Infectious Agents
    cytomegalovirus
    herpes hominis type II virus
    rubella virus
    Treponema pallidum (syphilis)
    Toxoplasma gondii
    varicella virus

Drugs and Chemicals
    alcohol
    amniopterin, methyamniopterin (folate antagonists)
    androgenic hormones
    busulfan (alkylating agents)
    diethylstilbesterol (DES)
    isotretinoin
    lead
    lithium
    organic mercury compounds
    phenytoin
    polybrominated biphenyls (PBBs)
    polychlorinated biphenyls (PCBs)
    tetracyclines
    thalidomide
    trimethadione
    valproic acid
    warfarin (anticoagulant)

Physical Agents
    hyperthermia
    ionizing radiation

the infection will be more devastating, but overall, fewer fetuses will be affected. On the other hand, if the infection occurs later, more fetuses will be infected, but the results may be relatively benign. In general, virus infections lead to central nervous damage, cardiac defects, and structural abnormalities in the fetus. Prenatal testing is possible in many cases to help determine the mother's exposure and vulnerability to these infections. See Chapter 13 for a complete discussion of these considerations.

Physical Agents

Maternal hyperthermia (overheating) leading to significant elevation of the temperature in the fetal compartment has been associated in animal studies with abnormalities when occurring during the period of organogenesis. Therefore, it is recommended that pregnant women avoid elevation of their body temperatures as may occur with excessive exposure to hot tubs and steam baths during the first trimester. It is also wise to monitor the body temperature during exercise, as discussed in the preceding chapter.

Radiation is another physical agent known to be responsible for fetal developmental defects. Studies of atomic bomb survivors in Japan have shown that fetal exposure to acute, high doses of radiation has led to an increased risk for mental and physical growth retardation. In comparison, the exposure to radiation from diagnostic tests, such as simple X rays, is significantly less risky. No proven ill effects have been reported at doses of less than twenty-five rads, although it is customary to limit exposure to five rads whenever possible during pregnancy. Then, if an X ray is necessary during pregnancy for evaluation of a potentially serious condition, it can usually be safely performed using abdominal shielding. Rad levels are cumulative, but with abdominal shielding, simple X-ray studies (chest, extremity, teeth) supply much less than one rad to the abdomen.

Environmental Agents

The pregnant or soon-to-be pregnant woman should be alert to a number of potentially harmful environmental factors. One of these is lead, which is found in the air, water, and soil; it is absorbed into our bodies from the air we breathe and from the food we eat. Excessive exposure to environmental lead can be harmful to anyone. In pregnant women, high levels of lead in maternal serum can lead to increased rates of spontaneous abortion, low birth weight, and infant developmental disabilities.

There are two main sources of environmental lead contamination besides industrial waste. These are lead paint and the combustion of leaded gasolines. In paint made before World War II, lead carbonate and lead oxide were common ingredients. The paint dust or chips have been eaten by children and can be inhaled. Lesser sources of lead include improperly glazed food containers and soluble lead compounds from lead plumbing pipes. Exposure to lead has decreased markedly since World War II. Leaded gasoline has been phased out, and the amount of lead in paint cannot exceed 1 percent. Workers who are still at risk are those employed in lead smelters and in storage battery factories and employees in pre–World War II buildings that have not been updated or that still have lead pipes. If you are concerned about your work surroundings, inquiries regarding lead levels in drinking water, air lead levels, and environmental safety should be addressed first to the building management. Further questions should be referred to the environmental safety office of your city or state government.

Lead is a neurotoxin and easily crosses the placenta.

Therefore, a woman should not work in an environment with air lead concentrations reaching 50 micrograms per cubic centimeter. Also, the level of lead in her blood should not be elevated. Lead accumulates within bone and can be mobilized long after excessive environmental exposure has ceased. Any woman planning pregnancy who may have had a previously high exposure to lead should have her serum levels checked on a regular basis to detect potential toxicity; this can be done at her physician's office or at a local hospital.

The organic environmental pollutants, primarily methylmercury, have been shown to be teratogenic in humans. Although methylmercury was previously used as a fungicide in the United States in the 1960s, our current exposure comes primarily from eating fish that have themselves become contaminated by eating food with a high mercury content. Organic mercury enters the food chain through industrial production, organic fuel exhaust, and pesticides.

The U.S. fishing industry imposes strict controls on the fish that go to market. They are routinely tested for mercury levels. Also, the Food and Drug Administration (FDA) randomly tests fish from across the country. In general, eating fish supplied by major distributors poses little risk. However, eating fish that have been caught by private individuals, and thus not subjected to testing, may be hazardous.

Mercury is slowly excreted from the body and can be measured in the system for longer than 120 days after the exposure. The compound easily crosses the placenta and accumulates in fetal brain tissue, where it significantly affects development. Methylmercury does not appear to cause structural defects in humans, and the problems associated with exposure may not show up in the newborn for months or years.

Polychlorinated biphenyls (PCBs) and polybrominated biphenyls (PBBs) were introduced into the environment by industry. They resist biodegradation and are highly lipid (fat) soluble. Therefore, they accumulate in fat tissue and breast milk in high concentrations. At present, the route of human exposure is primarily through eating fish from contaminated waters. High levels of these compounds have led to skin discoloration, tooth and gum abnormalities, bone changes, eye abnormalities, and growth retardation in a small number of exposed newborns.

Prescription and Over-the-Counter Medications

Many patients have questions regarding the safety of commonly used prescription and nonprescription medications during pregnancy. While these drugs are not teratogenic in the sense that they have been proven to cause structural abnormalities in exposed human fetuses, they may be responsible for causing other types of problems in pregnancy. Therefore, it is critical to stress that in pregnancy, *no drug, even over-the-counter medications, should be taken without the advice and consent of the treating physician.* This having been said, in the following paragraphs we review what is currently known about a number of commonly used medications. In reading this, bear in mind that no drug is known to be without effect in pregnancy, and some that we believe at the present time to be benign may prove to be dangerous later.

The most frequently recommended pain medication that can be purchased without a prescription is acetaminophen. No special risks are associated with it in pregnancy when used as directed. Aspirin and similar drugs such as ibuprofen are not recommended in pregnancy because their use has been associated with bleeding disorders in the mother and fetus due to platelet dysfunction, and detrimental cardiovascular changes in the fetus. However, certain drugs in this category have been successfully used as a treatment for premature labor and may be indicated in instances when prescribed and monitored by a physician.

Several nonprescription cough remedies appear to be safe for use in pregnancy. These include dextromethorphan, guaifenesin, and cetylpyridinium chloride; although others may be safe and beneficial, these are the drugs with which we have the most experience. We recommend that pregnant patients avoid cough medicines that contain potassium iodide, since this drug may be taken up by the fetal thyroid, causing goiter (enlargement).

When necessary, pseudoephedrine is commonly recommended by obstetricians as a decongestant, while medicines containing phenylpropanolamine and epinephrine should be avoided. They have been associated with an increased incidence of congenital defects in some studies.

Chlorpheniramine is the most commonly used antihistamine (antiallergy medicine) in pregnancy; most antihistamines are probably safe, based upon present available data. However, brompheniramine has been shown to be associated with an increased risk for malformations and should be avoided when pregnancy is suspected.

No pregnancy-related complications have yet been documented with the use of topical nasal sprays. The ones most commonly employed are the short-acting compound phenylephrine and the long-acting drug oxymetazoline.

Aminopterin and its derivatives are primarily chemotherapeutic agents for the treatment of cancer. These drugs act by inhibiting folic acid (folate) and should be avoided during pregnancy. Similarly, the alkylating agents such as busulfan, which are also chemotherapeutic agents for cancer therapy, should be avoided during gestation. However, in the rare circumstance in which a mother is diagnosed during pregnancy as having cancer, some chemotherapeutic agents may be indicated if the potential benefit to the mother is thought to outweigh the risk to the fetus.

Hormones, especially those with masculinizing effects,

can cause fetal damage. Generally, some of the synthetic forms of these hormones are the culprits. Natural hormones, such as progesterone, are considered safe, whereas some synthetic progestins (19-nortestosterone derivatives) can masculinize the female fetus. A synthetic estrogen, diethylstilbesterol, or DES, was unfortunately used for years as a treatment for threatened abortion during the first trimester of pregnancy. Many male and female fetuses were exposed, and they later suffered significant consequences, including an increased risk for certain types of cancer and reproductive disorders.

The birth control pill is the most commonly prescribed source of synthetic hormones, but even in cases where the pill has been continued inadvertently into the first trimester, fetal problems are extremely rare. Patients with certain infertility problems (luteal phase defect, for example) may be prescribed a progestational agent. However, the most commonly used hormone in this situation is the natural form of progesterone, which is not known to cause any fetal defects. Patients who are treated with danazol for endometriosis should stop the drug before conception. Danazol is a synthetic androgen (male) hormone and can cause masculinization of a female fetus.

Warfarin (Coumadin) is known to cause morphologic and developmental defects in the newborns of women treated with this drug. It is commonly used in the nonpregnant state to treat thrombosis or blood-clotting abnormalities. The fetal syndrome attributed to Coumadin use includes poor nasal growth, bone changes, optic abnormalities, and mental retardation. Women who require anticoagulation during pregnancy are best maintained on another drug, heparin. Heparin is safe in pregnancy because it does not cross the placenta.

The drug isotretinoin, commonly known as Accutane, has been marketed as a treatment for severe acne; typically, it is prescribed for teenagers. Some pregnancies have occurred inadvertently in this group, and about 25 percent have resulted in live-born fetuses with malformations. The abnormalities have been serious and have included hydrocephalus, small ears, and heart defects. Accutane is a derivative of vitamin A, which itself can be harmful if taken in doses significantly exceeding recommendation. These drugs are known to persist in storage form within the body for months or even years. Patients who anticipate pregnancy after the use of Accutane should consult their physician about the interval of time required before pregnancy can be safely undertaken.

A common concern centers upon the length of time one should wait to become pregnant after stopping oral contraceptives. Unlike Accutane and other derivatives of vitamin A, oral contraceptives do not have a residual effect, so it is probably unnecessary to postpone pregnancy after discontinuing their use.

Medications used in the treatment of epilepsy have been implicated in abnormal fetal development. Trimethadione and valproic acid should be avoided altogether in pregnancy whenever possible. However, the drug phenytoin, or Dilantin, is used in pregnancy to control seizures when necessary. Dilantin is associated with structural defects in a small percentage of exposed pregnancies. The fetal syndrome consists of a small head, growth deficiency, developmental delays, mental retardation, and changes in facial structure.

The well-known antibiotic tetracycline, which is commonly prescribed in the nonpregnant state for a variety of infections, should be avoided in pregnancy and early childhood, but if given prior to twelve weeks gestation it is unlikely to cause abnormalities. The drug causes a brownish discoloration of the teeth of the newborn and inhibits bone growth. Most of the effects of this drug are reversible with time.

Risk Factors for Commonly Used Medications

Health professionals, pharmaceutical manufacturers, and the FDA have come to a general consensus about the assignment of potential risk to the fetus from the most commonly used medications. Medications are assigned a risk category of A, B, C, D, or X depending upon the data available regarding safety in pregnancy. These categories are defined by the FDA as follows:

Category A. Controlled studies in women fail to demonstrate a risk to the fetus in the first trimester (and there is no evidence of a risk in later trimesters), and the possibility of harm appears remote.

Category B. Either animal-reproductive studies have not demonstrated a fetal risk but there are no controlled studies in pregnant women, or animal-reproductive studies have shown adverse effect (other than decreased fertility) that was not confirmed in controlled studies in women in the first trimester or any other trimester.

Category C. Either studies in animals have revealed adverse effects on the fetus (teratogenic or other) and there are not controlled studies in women, or studies in women and animals are not available. Drugs should be given only if the potential benefit justifies the potential risk to the fetus.

Category D. There is positive evidence of human fetal risk, but the benefits from use in pregnant women may be acceptable, despite the risk (e.g., if the drug is needed in a life-threatening situation or for a serious disease for which safer drugs cannot be used or are ineffective).

Category X. Studies in animals or human beings have demonstrated fetal abnormalities or there is evidence of fetal risk based on human experience or both, and the risk of the use of the drug in pregnant women clearly outweighs any possible benefit. The drug is contraindicated in women who are or may become pregnant.

The risk categories of some commonly used drugs are shown in Table 9-2. It should be emphasized that not all

TABLE 9-2

RISK CATEGORIES FOR COMMONLY USED MEDICATIONS

Drug	Use	Risk Category
acetaminophen	pain reliever	B
ampicillin	antibiotic	B
aspirin	pain reliever	C
cimetidine	ulcer medication	B
clomiphene	ovulation induction	X
cocaine	recreational drug, pain reliever	C
codeine	pain reliever	C
Coumadin	blood thinner	D
diazepam	tranquilizer	D
digitalis	heart medication	C
doxycycline	antibiotic	D
erythromycin	antibiotic	B
folic acid	nutrient	A
gentamicin	antibiotic	C
lithium	mood disorder medication	D
methadone	heroin substitute	B
metronidazole	antibiotic	B
morphine	pain reliever	B
nystatin	antifungal medication	B
penicillin	antibiotic	B
phenytoin	seizure medication	D
valproic acid	seizure medication	D
vitamin A	nutrient	A/X*

*In recommended dosages the category is A; in megadoses the category is X.

teratogens are X, and even drugs in the C or D categories may be indicated in pregnancy under certain circumstances. Your physician should review the risks and benefits of all medications prescribed during your pregnancy. As stated earlier, over-the-counter medications should be avoided in pregnancy unless you have consulted your physician.

The risk category to which a drug has been assigned can be determined from the *Physicians' Desk Reference*. However, not all drugs have been assigned to a category by their manufacturers. In such cases, the book *Drugs in Pregnancy and Lactation: A Reference Guide to Fetal and Neonatal Risk* by G. G. Briggs et al. (1983) can be consulted.

Recreational Drugs

Recreational drugs are known to have detrimental effects on pregnancy. Heroin users are at risk for intrauterine growth retardation, preterm birth, hepatitis, and AIDS. Their newborns usually suffer severe withdrawal reactions postpartum as a manifestation of their passive drug dependence. These reactions can be life-threatening if not recognized and appropriately treated in time. We recommend that pregnant women addicted to heroin be enrolled in a methadone maintenance program and not be allowed to withdraw during pregnancy. Methadone is an oral substitute for heroin which is provided for addicts through special programs. Complete withdrawal without methadone support can be dangerous for both mother and fetus during pregnancy.

The use of cocaine has skyrocketed in the last decade. Expectant mothers who use cocaine may suffer many pregnancy complications. The development of distress in labor is more likely among cocaine-exposed fetuses than among normal fetuses. Placental abruption, or hemorrhage behind the placenta, leading to premature separation of the placenta from the uterine wall, appears to be associated with the use of cocaine. Intrauterine growth retardation is also more likely in these newborns; cocaine causes the placental vessels to constrict, thus decreasing the oxygen supply to the fetus.

Approximately 14 percent of pregnant women admit to using marijuana, and the true percentage of users may be significantly higher. Although birth defects (malformations) are not believed to be associated with marijuana use, premature births probably occur more frequently in the pregnancies of heavy users. Newborns who have been exposed to marijuana in utero demonstrate slow or delayed startle responses in the early postpartum period. This appears to resolve with time, but adequate long-term follow-up studies are lacking. Clearly, recreational drug use must be eliminated during pregnancy to ensure the safety of both the mother and the fetus.

Alcohol, Caffeine, Cigarettes

Alcohol, as do the majority of teratogenic agents, easily crosses the placenta. The adverse effects of alcohol on pregnancy have been reported since at least 1973. The first studies described what is termed fetal alcohol syndrome in infants of alcoholic mothers. The disorder includes central nervous system dysfunction, mental retardation, small head and lower jaw size, and other distinctive ocular, facial, and skeletal disorders. The incidence of the full-blown syndrome is low, even in alcoholic mothers, but milder forms occur in a significant number of pregnancies when high alcohol intake is a factor. Some reviews report that mothers must have three drinks a day before the risk of effect is significantly increased, but other studies suggest that no level of drinking is completely safe.

My advice to women seeking pregnancy is this: Stop drinking when pregnancy is planned, especially since weeks two to eight after conception are so critical for proper development. Because we do not know if there is a "safe" limit for alcohol consumption during pregnancy, abstinence is best. A woman should stop drinking before conception; alcohol present at discrete times during embryogenesis can cause fetal alcohol syndrome.

A few studies have described complications in the pregnancies of women who consume large amounts of caffeine (the equivalent of four cups of coffee per day or more — about 400 milligrams of caffeine per day). Although the findings are controversial and not confirmed by all studies, there may be an increased risk for intrauterine growth retardation or late first trimester spontaneous abortion (miscarriage) in these women. We recommend that pregnant women limit their caffeine intake or avoid caffeine altogether whenever possible. However, there is no evidence for an increased incidence of congenital malformations (birth defects) as a result of caffeine.

Tobacco smoke is not included on the list of known human teratogens, but it has many detrimental effects on pregnancy. Mothers who smoke have an increased risk for spontaneous first trimester pregnancy loss, premature labor, premature rupture of the membranes, third trimester bleeding, and fetal growth retardation leading to low birth weight!

Cigarette smoke contains thousands of different compounds, many of which are not well characterized. We believe that the compounds that act to deprive the fetus of its oxygen supply cause the most harm. The worst offenders are probably nicotine, carbon monoxide, and cyanide. Nicotine causes constriction, or narrowing, of the walls of the placental blood vessels. This can result in a more than 20 percent decrease in placental blood flow. Carbon monoxide displaces oxygen from hemoglobin, which carries oxygen in the blood to the tissues. Thus, less oxygen is available for delivery to the tissues. The capacity of carbon monoxide to displace oxygen is even greater in the fetus. Fetal hemoglobin is modified to have less affinity for oxygen than adult hemoglobin. Therefore, the effects of carbon monoxide are magnified in the fetus. Cyanide is toxic to growing tissues, and nutrients that are needed elsewhere for growth (vitamin B_{12}, amino acids) must be diverted to break down cyanide. Thus, chronic exposure to cyanide can lead to intrauterine growth retardation.

In addition to the long list of pregnancy complications associated with smoking, evidence is mounting that children of smoking parents may be at risk for growth and developmental delays as children. There is some medical evidence to suggest that sudden infant death syndrome (SIDS) is increased in these babies. Also, respiratory ailments are more commonly seen in the children of smokers. In older children, physical growth may be stunted and behavioral problems such as hyperactivity may occur more frequently. Studies indicate that "passive" smoking (mother inhaling someone else's smoke) during pregnancy can result in low birth weight. For all these reasons, as well as for the health of the parents, we would strongly suggest that the prospective mother and father quit smoking before conception.

[PART IV]

Marking Progress, Detecting Complications: Tests Before and During Pregnancy

[10]

The Pap Smear
Luis E. Sanz, M.D.

*The Papanicolaou smear is an integral part of almost all gyne-
cologic exams and is usually performed on the first visit to the
obstetrician's office during pregnancy. This simple test truly
should be part of preparation for pregnancy. Clinical situations
that might pose all sorts of difficulties in evaluation and treatment
if detected during pregnancy can be dealt with easily if detected
before pregnancy. The physician gently scrapes surface cells off
the outside of the cervix and cervical canal to look for potential
changes that might produce cervical cancer in the future if left
untreated. Most cancers of the cervix take years to develop. Early
detection of premalignant changes in the cervical cells allows the
opportunity for treatment, which can prevent the development
of cancer. The treatment involves destroying the abnormal tissue
by heat, laser, freezing, or chemicals. In more severe cases, it
may be necessary to surgically remove the tissue, a procedure
called a cone biopsy.*

*It has been three decades since Dr. George Papanicolaou de-
veloped this testing technique. Since then, many thousands of
women have been saved from death because of early cancer
detection. We believe that it is very important for all women to*

understand the Pap smear so that cervical abnormalities can be detected in the premalignant phase. In addition to detecting premalignant changes in the cervix, the Pap test provides other valuable information. For example, the presence of some vaginal infections can be diagnosed by Pap smear. It also gives some indication of hormonal levels. As you read this chapter, you will see how this test provides much information for continuing good health care.

HAVE YOU EVER wondered why there is such an emphasis placed on Pap smears? Did you ever question what might happen should a Pap smear be read as abnormal? You probably know that the test has something to do with cancer, but exactly what might have evaded you. The following discussion will help you understand the implications of this test and will explain the workup that accompanies an abnormal reading.

The Pap smear is a simple screening test. It is easy to perform and has become a routine test in periodic health exams of women. It serves as a warning flag, indicating to the physician when abnormal changes leading to cancer may be occurring in the cervix. Its beauty lies in its simplicity and in the fact that when read as abnormal, it is rarely wrong. Unfortunately, it does carry with it a 15 to 40 percent false-negative rate, that is, something serious may be occurring and the test will still be read as normal. Routine Pap smears give doctors the ability to detect abnormal changes in the cervix before they become cancerous or symptomatic. The progression from early abnormal cell changes to cervical cancer usually occurs over several years. When detected early enough, the problem is completely curable!

In order to understand the medical workup that accompanies an abnormal Pap test, one must have an appreciation for the cellular changes that occur naturally and in disease states in the cervix.

In a woman's early life, the cervix is completely covered by a thin layer of columnar cells. These are relatively fragile, and through a natural process, many are replaced by harder, flatter, squamous (scalelike) cells. This transition occurs at the end of the cervix, the portion closest to the vagina, in the area known as the transformation zone (T-zone). The process is called squamous metaplasia. Cancer of the cervix arises in the T-zone. Therefore, it is from this area that the Pap smear is obtained.

When cells undergo malignant changes, they alter in appearance. A pathologist can detect these changes using special stains under microscopic examination. Before becoming malignant, cells will pass through a state known as dysplasia. They may be large, irregular in shape, and have peculiar nuclei (the "brain" of the cell). Cancer cells become even more bizarre and multiply uncontrollably.

Five divisions were employed in the original classification system set up by Dr. Papanicolaou. This system was used for many years and served as the basis for more modern revisions. Class I meant that normal cells were seen. Class V indicated that definite malignant cells were present on the slide. The middle classes II through IV were used to describe atypical cells and those cells that were suggestive or highly suggestive of malignancy.

Revisions of the original pap smear classifications have stressed descriptive terms instead of just numbers to give the doctor a clearer understanding of the disease and appropriate treatment. Infections such as trichomonas, herpes, and yeast organisms are specified on the report if identified under the microscope. The newer terminology also takes into account the progressive nature of premalignant disease of the cervix as well as the important association of the human papillomavirus with regard to cervical cancer and its precursors. A comparison table (10-1) lists the Papanicolaou classification and the latest revision by the National Cancer Institute in December of 1988.

Finding atypical cells on a pap smear is a very common occurrence. The physician will reevaluate the patient in regard to cervical infection and generally repeat the pap smear. If the patient has any suggestive findings of the papillomavirus, a history of previous cervical disease, or a partner with genital warts, a colposcopic examination may be performed after just one atypical pap smear. A low-powered microscope known as the colposcope is used by the gynecologist to observe the transformation zone of the cervix directly. The trained eye will be able to detect changes on the surface of the cervix that indicate premalignant disease. Using the colposcope as a guide, a small punch biopsy of the abnormal area is obtained. Scrapings of the cervical canal (endocervical curettage, ECC) may

TABLE 10-1
CLASSIFICATION OF PAP SMEARS

	Papanicolaou	Proposed Revision
I	No evidence of malignancy	Within normal limits
II	Atypical cells	Atypical cells
III	Suggestive of malignancy	Low-grade lesion (includes early papillomavirus lesions and mild dysplasia)
IV	Strongly suggestive of malignancy	High-grade lesion (includes more severe premalignant lesions of the cervix that have not yet invaded)
V	Conclusive for malignancy	Squamous carcinoma

also be taken. The pathologist is then able to examine the biopsies and determine the extent of disease so that appropriate therapy may be given. The punch biopsy and ECC may cause brief pinching pain or cramping but do not require anesthesia.

If the colposcopy and biopsies do not provide enough information to explain the initial abnormal Pap smear, a cone biopsy is necessary. Under general anesthesia, a cone-shaped area that incorporates tissue from the T-zone is excised. The surgeon does this by cutting a wedge-shaped piece of tissue (approximately one inch in diameter at its widest part) from the cervix. It too is sent for pathological evaluation. Cone biopsies may be done as outpatient surgery or may require overnight hospitalization. Although the procedure is relatively simple, it does carry some risks of bleeding and infection.

All of the biopsies obtained are evaluated in terms of the severity and extent of cervical disease. Appropriate therapy is then selected.

Dysplasia, cellular changes that are considered premalignant, may be treated with cryosurgery, laser therapy, or cone biopsy. Cryosurgery is a simple office procedure whereby the cells of the cervix in the area of the transformation zone are frozen and thus die. Laser therapy is a concentrated beam of light used to destroy the precancerous cells. Cone biopsy is also a way of surgically removing diseased tissue.

Invasive cancer of the cervix obviously requires more extensive therapy. Depending on the extent of disease, radical hysterectomy (surgical removal of the uterus, cervix, and associated lymph nodes) or radiotherapy may be required. Fortunately, the use of Pap smears as a screening technique has markedly decreased the occurrence of cancer of the cervix.

[11]

Genetics and Genetic Counseling

L. Pat Robinson, M.D.

You probably know a lot more about genetics than you think. For instance, you know that height, eye color, and baldness are hereditary traits. Yet, many people are intimidated by the subject of genetics, fearing that it is too complicated to understand. This really is not so, and the genetic information that is pertinent for most couples is relatively easy to understand. The most important thing is to know whether you are at risk for a genetic problem, and if so, just what the extent of the risk is. In this chapter, Dr. Robinson presents an overview of the elements of genetic counseling as they relate to pregnancy.

MOST PARENTS have healthy babies, yet every couple faces the risk of birth defects in their child. Most defects are relatively minor, such as an extra finger or toe (called polydactyly); some are major, such as heart defects or spina bifida. The basic, or background, risk — that is, the random risk that any couple faces — of having a child with a birth defect is about 3 percent (3 in every 100 births). The cause for most of these defects is not well understood, and most cannot be identified before the birth of the affected child. However, some couples, because of their medical history, their family history, the mother's age, or the couple's ethnic origin, face a risk greater than the background risk of having a child with a birth defect. For these couples, genetic counseling is especially informative and helpful in decision-making.

Who Needs Genetic Counseling, and How Can It Help?

Couples are usually referred to a geneticist by a family physician, internist, or obstetrician. Reporting a complete and accurate personal and family history to your primary-care physician will help to determine if you may be at increased risk. Common indicators that genetic counseling is needed are:

- Maternal age over thirty-four at the time of delivery.
- Previous child with a chromosome disorder.
- Couples who have had two or more spontaneous abortions (miscarriages).
- Parent or close family member with a chromosome abnormality.
- Personal or family history of a genetic disease, mental retardation, or birth defect (includes parents).
- Mother and father both carriers of a recessive gene (such as Tay-Sachs or sickle cell).
- Mother carrier of an X-linked recessive gene (such as hemophilia, Duchenne muscular dystrophy).
- Previous child with a birth defect or neonatal death of unknown cause.
- Previous child with spina bifida or anencephaly (types of neural tube defects).
- Marriage between related individuals (consanguinity).
- Maternal disease affecting pregnancy (diabetes mellitus, lupus erythematosus, seizure disorders).

Most individuals at increased risk are identified by their age or reproductive history. Other factors, such as infertility or recurrent abortions, may prompt chromosome testing and identify carriers of chromosome abnormalities. A family history of an X-linked disease in the brother, maternal uncle, or nephew of a woman may place her at risk to be a carrier for one of these abnormal genes. In most cases, specific blood tests can determine if an individual is at increased risk or not.

If your family history indicates a need for it, genetic counseling can help to identify whether you are in fact at increased risk to have a child with a problem and can provide information about what can be done. During genetic counseling, you will learn what your special risk is, information about the condition you may be at risk for, and ways to predict a problem and in some cases how to prevent or treat it.

Genetic counseling is an educational process based on an exchange of information between you and a geneticist — a specially trained counselor, nurse, social worker, scientist, or physician — who will start by collecting detailed medical information from you. The information will include a carefully taken family medical history that enables the counselor to create a family tree, or pedigree, showing the relationship between individuals. Sometimes blood or tissue tests to study genetic material are needed. The result of this evaluation allows the counselor to assess the risk that you will develop a genetic or familial condition or will have a child born with such a condition.

After relaying this risk assessment to you, the counselor will explain the prepregnancy and prenatal predictive tests that are available and outline their risks, benefits, and accuracy. He or she will then assist you in deciding what steps to take next. Exploring the possible need for genetic counseling should ideally be part of every couple's prepregnancy planning. Early detection of potential problems will allow you time to make reasoned, responsible decisions.

Types of Genetic Diseases

As a background to understanding how certain kinds of diseases or defects may be inherited, it may be helpful to review some of the basics of genetics.

The genetic material of a cell is the blueprint or instruction for cell function. Each body cell contains forty-six pieces of genetic material called chromosomes, arranged in twenty-three pairs — twenty-two "regular" chromosome pairs and one pair that determines sex. In a male, the sex chromosome pair is made up of one X chromosome and one Y chromosome; a female has two copies of the X chromosome. One of the members of each pair of chromosomes was inherited from the mother and the other member of the pair from the father. When a man makes sperm and a woman makes an egg, each developing sperm or egg gets one member of each chromosome pair, exactly twenty-three chromosomes. When the sperm fertilizes the egg, the resulting normal conception thus has forty-six chromosomes. All of a woman's eggs normally contain one X chromosome; half of a male's sperm are X-bearing and half are Y-bearing. The father's sperm, then, determines the sex of the child, depending on whether the egg is fertilized by an X-bearing sperm, resulting in a female, or a Y-bearing sperm, resulting in a male. Normal development requires forty-six chromosomes. Extra or missing chromosomal material leads to developmental abnormalities, some of which are discussed below.

Each chromosome is composed of deoxyribonucleic acid (DNA), which is made up of many units of genetic information called genes. The way a gene expresses itself determines how it is inherited. The two members of a pair of chromosomes have corresponding but not exactly identical genetic information. A dominant gene need be present in only one copy, or one of the members of a pair, to express its effect. For example, a child who inherits one gene for brown hair and one for red hair will have brown hair because the gene for brown hair is dominant. A recessive gene requires that two copies of the gene be present, one on each member of the pair, for its effect to be seen. Red hair is inherited via a recessive gene, so in order to have red hair, a child must inherit the gene from both parents.

Certain abnormal recessive genes carried on the X chromosome, however, need be present in only one copy to manifest themselves if the gene is inherited by a male. This is because males have only one X chromosome and the Y chromosome lacks a normal gene to offset the abnormal X-linked gene. A female with an abnormal X-linked recessive gene has a second X chromosome with a normal dominant gene and thus will not show the effect of the abnormal gene; she may, however, pass the abnormal gene to her offspring. Hemophilia, a blood-clotting defect, is an X-linked disease. A woman who carries the abnormal gene will not be a hemophiliac; but if her son inherits the gene he will suffer the disease.

Genetic diseases can be classified into three main groups based on their cause: chromosome disorders, single-gene disorders, and multifactorial diseases.

Chromosome Disorders

A chromosome disorder is present whenever there is more or less than the normal number of chromosomes or when a piece of chromosome material is missing, duplicated, or rearranged. The problems observed vary depending on the specific chromosome disorder present. Extra or missing chromosome material almost always results in serious birth

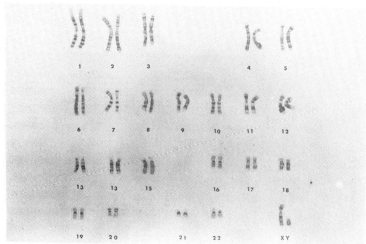

Figure 11-1. Normal Male Karyotype. There are twenty-three pairs of chromosomes arranged by size, shape, and banding (G-bands in this figure). The first twenty-two pairs are called autosomes. The twenty-third pair comprises sex chromosomes, the X and smaller Y chromosomes connoting a normal male. (Karotypes courtesy of Dr. Avirachan Tharapel and Dr. Joe Leigh Simpson, University of Tennessee, Memphis.)

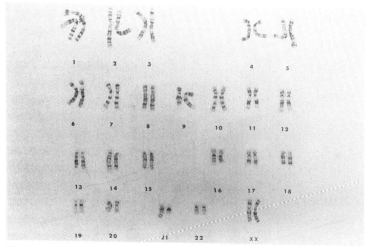

Figure 11-2. Normal Female Karyotype. There are twenty-two pairs of autosomes. The twenty-third pair contains two X chromosomes, connoting a normal female karyotype.

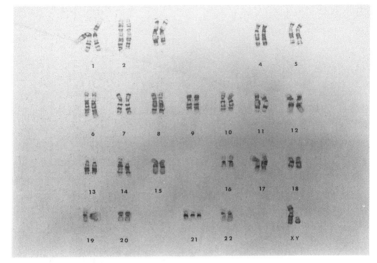

Figure 11-3. Trisomy 21 Karyotype (Down Syndrome). There are forty-seven chromosomes due to an extra number 21 chromosome. The twenty-third pair contains an X and Y chromosome, indicating that there is a male fetus with Down syndrome.

defects or mental retardation. Rearrangement of chromosome material, without loss or gain of DNA, does not affect appearance, mentation, or development, but it does increase the chance of conceiving a child with a chromosome abnormality and increases the chances of recurrent spontaneous abortion. Overall, 1 in every 160 babies is born with a chromosome problem.

Down syndrome is a common chromosome disorder and is caused in 96 percent of cases by the presence of an extra copy of chromosome number 21. Down syndrome affects 1 in 700 newborns and results in a characteristic facial appearance and varying degrees of mental retardation. Cardiac and intestinal manifestations are common as well. Even more severe growth and mental retardation occurs when the extra chromosome is number 13 or number 18.

On the other hand, abnormalities in the number of sex

chromosomes may result in much milder problems. A female with a missing X chromosome (Turner syndrome) will be short and infertile and may have cardiac and kidney defects, but is usually of average intelligence. An extra X chromosome in a male (Klinefelter syndrome) may manifest itself only in infertility; however, some XXY males have more serious problems with sexual maturation and psychological development.

Four groups of people are at increased risk to have a child born with a chromosome problem:

• Every couple has some risk of having a child born with an extra chromosome, but the risk increases as the mother's age at the time of delivery increases (see Table 11-1). There is no absolute cutoff for concern, but general recommendations are that a woman aged thirty-four or thirty-five at the time of delivery be referred for genetic counseling. A younger woman who is concerned about her risk may elect to have counseling too. During the counseling session, the risks and benefits of prenatal diagnosis to identify a fetus with a chromosome abnormality will be explained to the

TABLE 11-1
MATERNAL AGE AND CHROMOSOME ABNORMALITIES
IN NEWBORNS

Maternal Age	Risk of Down Syndrome	Risk for All Chromosome Abnormalities
20	1/1600	1/475
25	1/1200	1/475
30	1/950	1/385
35	1/385	1/200
40	1/100	1/60
45	1/30	1/20

E. B. Hook, "Rates of Chromosome Abnormalities at Different Maternal Ages," *Obstetrics and Gynecology* 58 (1981), 282–285.

couple. The decision to have fetal testing is up to the woman at risk. The tests available to study the fetal chromosomal characteristics include chorionic villus sampling and amniocentesis (see below) and can only be performed during pregnancy.

• Couples who have had a prior child with a chromosome abnormality are at higher risk than the background risk to have the problem recur.

• A physically normal parent who has a chromosome abnormality is at increased risk to have a child with a chromosome problem. Such a parent may be identified when a chromosome study is performed to evaluate infertility, amenorrhea (absent menses), or recurrent early pregnancy losses.

• Individuals with close relatives who have chromosome abnormalities or certain types of mental retardation may also be carriers of hidden chromosome abnormalities. For example, about 2 to 3 percent of Down syndrome cases are caused by a translocation of a copy of chromosome number 21 to another chromosome. This "familial" type of Down syndrome may have been inherited from a normal-appearing parent who has a rearrangement of his or her chromosomes. Other family members may also be carriers of this translocation, which only manifests itself in increased risk for pregnancy loss and children with chromosome abnormalities. Many such types of chromosome rearrangements occur. Chromosome testing of the affected individual, or in some cases other family members, can clarify the risks for the family.

SINGLE-GENE DISORDERS

As we have seen, each chromosome is made up of many genes, which are the units of genetic information. Diseases caused by gene defects are grouped based on their function and behavior. Dominant abnormal genes show their effect when present in one copy, that is, when present in only one of a pair of chromosomes; recessive abnormal genes require two copies, one on each member of the pair, to show their effect. An individual with one copy of a recessive gene is called a carrier and does not generally show the effect of the recessive gene. X-linked genes are carried on the X chromosome and manifest their effect in males.

Three groups of people are at increased risk to have a child born with a single-gene problem.

• If one member of a couple has a dominant inherited genetic disease, that parent has a 1 in 2 chance of passing the gene to their child.

• Parents who are both carriers for an abnormal recessive gene are at a 1 in 4 (25 percent) risk to have an affected child. For some recessive diseases, parents are identified as carriers only after they have given birth to an affected child. For example, cystic fibrosis is a recessively inherited disease; it causes both lung and intestinal problems and requires frequent hospitalizations for infections. At present, no test is available to identify carriers for the gene for cystic fibrosis before an affected child is born in a family. However, family members at risk to be carriers because of a known affected relative may be able to undergo DNA tests to find out which family members are carriers. For a few recessively inherited diseases, carrier testing is available before the birth of an affected child. Individuals are identified to be at risk to be carriers for these genes based on their ethnic background. Once one person in a family is found to be a carrier, other family members may consider testing as well (see Carrier Testing, below).

• A mother who is a carrier for an abnormal gene on the X chromosome is at risk to have sons affected with the disease. Abnormal genes located on the X chromosome include hemophilia A and B and Duchenne muscular dystrophy. Carriers are usually identified because of family history or after the birth of an affected child.

Other genetic disorders can be tested for by evaluating the function of the gene. These diagnostic tests, usually a protein analysis, are simple blood tests that typically require the affected family member to be tested. The test for the effect of the gene can be performed on a pregnancy at risk with cells obtained by amniocentesis or by chorionic villus sampling.

For a growing list of genetic diseases, DNA testing can identify an affected individual or carrier for an abnormal gene. For some diseases, DNA testing requires blood or tissue from the affected individual; for others, direct testing can be performed without such a comparison.

MULTIFACTORIAL DISEASES

Many common birth defects, including cleft lip (harelip), clubfoot, and congenital heart disease, are caused by a combination of both genetic and environmental factors. Because many factors are involved in their development, they are called multifactorial. Any couple can have a child born with a multifactorial birth defect. If a couple has a family history of a multifactorial birth defect, they may be at higher risk than the background risk.

Prevention of Birth Defects: Carrier Testing and Prenatal Diagnosis

For couples at risk, there are several options to choose from. The genetic counseling process helps families to make the choice that is most comfortable for them. Carrier tests for some diseases can identify couples at risk for recessive disorders before pregnancy. During pregnancy, several methods for prenatal diagnosis are available:

maternal serum alpha fetoprotein
ultrasound
amniocentesis
chorionic villus sampling
fetal blood sampling, skin or liver biopsy

Maternal serum alpha fetoprotein (MSAFP) and ultrasonography are useful screening tests. Amniocentesis and chorionic villus sampling are available to diagnose specific genetic disorders in the fetus. In rare instances, direct testing of the fetal blood or tissue may be indicated. Fortunately, in most cases the prenatal results from tests are normal, and a healthy baby can be anticipated.

CARRIER TESTING

Carrier tests are blood tests to identify hidden abnormal genes. A carrier is a healthy person with a pair of genes in which one is normal and one abnormal. If two carrier parents pass the abnormal genes to their child, the child will develop the disease. Individuals who may be at risk for a genetic disease are identified by their family history or by their ethnic background. If a disease is present in a family, tests may be available to identify which family members are carriers. For a few genetic diseases, testing is recommended based on ethnic background. Ashkenazi Jews are at risk for Tay-Sachs disease, a lethal disorder caused by storage of lipids in the central nervous system; blacks are at risk for sickle cell anemia; and individuals from the Mediterranean or Southeast Asia are potential carriers of thalassemia, another form of anemia. Most carrier tests are simple blood tests. Screening of at-risk groups by ethnic background can identify couples in which both persons are carriers and at risk even before conception.

TABLE 11-2
INDICATIONS FOR CARRIER TESTING

At-risk Group	Disease	Chance to Be a Carrier
Blacks	sickle cell anemia	1/10
Ashkenazi Jews	Tay-Sachs disease	1/30
Greeks, Italians	beta thalassemia	1/30
Southeast Asians, Chinese	alpha thalassemia	1/25

M. M. Kaback, "Heterozygote Screening," in A. E. Emery, *Principles and Practice of Medical Genetics*. Edinburgh: Churchill Livingstone, 1983.

Testing of the fetus during pregnancy can tell if the fetus is affected or not.

MATERNAL SERUM ALPHA FETOPROTEIN (MSAFP)
MSAFP is a screening test done on a blood sample obtained from the mother during the fifteenth to sixteenth week of pregnancy. The test measures a protein made by the fetus called alpha fetoprotein. All pregnant women have some of this protein in their blood. Some pregnancies tested will have too high or too low levels of MSAFP, but only a few of these pregnancies turn out to have serious problems. Other explanations for abnormal blood tests are often found, including the presence of twins or triplets or an error in determining the date of conception. When the level of the MSAFP is too high or too low, further testing is needed. The blood test may be repeated and an ultrasound ordered. If no other explanation for the abnormal result can be found, amniocentesis can be performed. Very low levels of MSAFP are associated with chromosome abnormalities in the fetus, and fetal chromosome studies can be tested on amniotic fluid. High levels are associated with anencephaly (easily detected by sonography) and fetal spina bifida. Analysis of amniotic fluid AFP and an addi-

tional protein called acetylcholinesterase, along with a careful ultrasound, can help to determine if the fetus has spina bifida. Only a few fetuses turn out to have problems, but most would not be identified without the use of MSAFP to screen the pregnancy.

ULTRASONOGRAPHY

Ultrasound, or sonography, creates a sound-wave picture of a pregnancy. The black-and-white image shows fetal movement, including fetal breathing and heart motion. Measurement of fetal growth can check the due date of the pregnancy. Twins and triplets can be identified, as well as the location of the placenta. Careful measurements of the length of the bones and study of the fetal heart, kidneys, stomach, and spine can detect many birth defects, though not all of the parts of the fetus can be studied, and not all birth defects can be identified. To the best of our knowledge, ultrasound is a safe procedure with no risk to the mother or fetus. (This important diagnostic tool is the subject of Chapter 15.)

AMNIOCENTESIS

Amniocentesis is usually done between fourteen and seventeen weeks of pregnancy. After an ultrasound locates the fetus and placenta, the physician directs a slender needle into the amniotic fluid. Usually, less than a tablespoon of fluid is removed. Fetal cells in the amniotic fluid can be used to test for several types of birth defects. Cytogenetic studies can identify Down syndrome or other chromosome abnormalities. Many single-gene disorders can be detected by testing for the specific defect or for the abnormal gene that causes the defect. The fetal sex can be determined from the chromosome studies as well. Results from amniocentesis are available from one to three weeks after testing.

The alpha fetoprotein can also be measured in amniotic

fluid. It is elevated when there is an opening somewhere in the fetal skin — such as spina bifida. AFP is measured in all amniotic fluid specimens, even if the pregnancy is not at increased risk, as a screening test for this group of abnormalities. Amniocentesis is a safe and accurate procedure but does involve some risk for the pregnancy. The risk that a pregnancy would miscarry because of the procedure is probably less than 0.5 percent, or less than 1 in 200. It may even be as low as 0.3 or 0.2 percent (1 in 300 or 1 in 500). Since the risk for a chromosome abnormality in the newborn is 1 in 320 when the mother is thirty-four, the benefit of fetal testing may outweigh the risk to the pregnancy. However, the perception of the risk and benefit of testing varies from individual to individual, and the decision to have the test or not will be up to the mother.

CHORIONIC VILLUS SAMPLING (CVS)
This test is used to sample cells from the developing placenta. The chromosome studies and single-gene tests done on amniotic fluid can also be done on these cells. The test is performed during the ninth to twelfth week of pregnancy. Guided by ultrasound, a thin tube is passed through the

TABLE 11-3
AMNIOCENTESIS OR CHORIONIC VILLUS SAMPLING

Maternal age over thirty-four at delivery
Previous child with a chromosome abnormality
Parents carriers for a recessive or dominant disease that can be
    tested for
Mother carrier for an X-linked disease
Previous child with a neural tube defect
Abnormally high or low maternal serum alpha fetoprotein
Abnormal ultrasound findings in the fetus
Pregnancy complications: growth delay in the fetus, too much or too
    little amniotic fluid

mother's cervix or a fine needle is inserted through the abdomen to the developing placenta and a piece of the placenta is aspirated. Results can be available within a few days to a week. This new test is comparable in safety and efficacy to amniocentesis. Problems with interpreting the results of the test lead to an amniocentesis in occasional patients. Nevertheless, the advantages of early testing and rapid results lead many patients to choose this test. An MSAFP must be done if screening for spina bifida is desired.

SPECIAL STUDIES

When the couple's family or reproductive history puts them at risk for a specific disease, special testing may be indicated. For diagnosis of a few very rare disorders, more invasive tests are required. For example, a specimen of fetal blood, muscle, liver, or skin may be needed. Sometimes a fetal X ray provides information about possible skeletal disorders. Fetal problems detected on an ultrasound may occasionally point to the need for chromosome studies on the fetus. Certain obstetric problems, such as fetal growth delay or too much or too little amniotic fluid, may also require amniocentesis for clarification.

Options

Most of the time, prenatal testing gives normal results. The couple can then be reassured that the fetus does not have the disorder it was tested for. However, some test results are abnormal. For these families, genetic counseling can provide information about the type of abnormality present and the effect it will have on the development of the child. Treatment is not available for the mental and growth retardation caused by chromosome diseases. For a few single-gene defects, medical therapy is helpful or curative, and surgery is available to treat many birth defects. The probable outcome after treatment can also be discussed with a genetic counselor and with other specialists.

Some couples decide to continue the pregnancy after a fetus with a problem has been detected. They may prepare for the birth of the affected child, or they may plan to place the child for adoption. Other couples decide to end the pregnancy. Both groups of parents may seek counseling help from geneticists, family, friends, clergy, and other professionals. The decision in all cases is a difficult one that the parents must make for themselves.

Prevention

After the diagnosis of an abnormal fetus, most couples choose to have prenatal testing for their next pregnancies. Fortunately, most couples face low recurrence risks, and chances are that their next pregnancy will be normal.

To avoid some problems, parents may choose an alternative means of conception. When couples are carriers for a recessive gene, or if one parent has a genetic disease or chromosome abnormality, the couple can elect to bypass this problem by using a sperm donor for artificial insemination or egg donor for in vitro fertilization. This alternative eliminates the risk that the parents will pass the problem to their child. Artificial insemination is relatively simple and inexpensive, but in vitro fertilization is a complicated, expensive procedure that is not always successful. A third choice for couples is adoption.

Not every couple needs genetic counseling. Most couples have healthy babies. For couples with a family history of a genetic disease or who suspect they may be at special risk, genetic counseling can provide accurate and usually reassuring information. Most major medical centers have genetic counseling clinics where expert advice, carrier testing, and prenatal diagnostic studies are available. Planning before pregnancy enables the counselors to collect information about the affected family members and determine if a couple faces special risk or not. Often, special blood studies require a lengthy time to complete. Planning before pregnancy allows time for the most accurate and careful information to be gathered for the parent-to-be.

[12]

Sexually Transmitted Diseases
Luis E. Sanz, M.D.

Conditions change rapidly in modern society. Just a few decades ago, a pregnant woman would be tested for syphilis at the beginning of her pregnancy and perhaps for gonorrhea if indicated. Today, many more venereal (sexually transmitted) diseases are commonly encountered; therefore, testing for some of these diseases must be considered a standard part of prepregnancy or prenatal care.

Perhaps you are not aware that chlamydia is now the most common venereal disease. Chlamydia is often asymptomatic, or without symptoms, so the mother may be totally unaware that she has this problem. The incidence of gonorrhea has remained the same over the years. The risk of syphilis is still present, and certainly one must consider the possibility of herpes. Trichomonas infections deserve mention. While they usually cause only vaginal irritation and discharge, their treatment during pregnancy can be problematic. All of these infections may sound like enormous threats. In actuality, the problem is not so formidable, but you should be aware that there will be more screening tests done in the doctor's office. Avoiding the complications that can result from venereal disease is another strong argument for following a program of preparation for pregnancy. Certainly, de-

tecting and eradicating such disease before the pregnancy improves the prospect of a good outcome. This chapter will present the common sexually transmitted diseases and attempt to give you some perspectives concerning these problems.

SEXUALLY TRANSMITTED DISEASES are extremely prevalent in our society. They know no sociologic or economic boundaries. While the advent of antibiotic therapy has provided cures for many of these diseases, changing sexual practices and increasing bacterial resistance to antibiotics contribute to their persistence. The importance of their diagnosis and treatment cannot be overemphasized, particularly to those preparing for pregnancy.

While many of the sexually transmitted diseases are relatively benign, certain ones are capable of causing more serious illness. Not only are infected adults at risk, but their fetuses can also suffer untoward effects. This chapter will focus on those sexually transmitted diseases pertinent to individuals preparing for pregnancy. Signs, symptoms, diagnosis, and treatment of these infections will be discussed.

Chlamydia

The organism *Chlamydia trachomatis* is capable of causing a wide variety of diseases. Of significance to the couple preparing for pregnancy are the facts that chlamydia infections can cause infertility in the woman and genital and eye infections in the newborn. In pregnancy, chlamydia has also been associated with premature rupture of the membranes and possibly premature labor.

Chlamydia is the most common sexually transmitted disease. In males, it often causes painful inflammation of the urethra. Like gonorrhea, it is capable of causing serious reproductive tract infections with subsequent scarring and infertility. In females, chlamydia may be asymptomatic and may only be detected by laboratory tests or cultures of the genital tract. However, it frequently causes inflammation of the urinary tract, vagina, and cervix. Chlamydia infections lead to increased infertility and likelihood of ectopic pregnancy (gestation outside the uterus), particularly if the infection has involved the fallopian tubes.

Chlamydia infections are effectively treated with tetracycline or erythromycin. In the pregnant patient, erythromycin is the drug of choice, and tetracycline is contraindicated because it can cause brown staining of the fetal teeth if used in the second half of pregnancy.

During the birth process, mothers with chlamydia infections may pass the organism to their children. If this happens, the newborn develops an eye infection known as inclusion conjunctivitis approximately one week after birth. An inflammation is the hallmark of this infection. It may occur in one or both eyes. Treatment requires a local antibiotic such as erythromycin.

Chlamydia trachomatis may also cause pneumonia in infants of infected mothers. Apparently, the respiratory tract becomes infected during birth. One to four months later, the child develops an atypical form of pneumonia. Fortunately, antibiotics are effective for treatment.

Gonorrhea

Gonorrhea is a bacterial disease that continues to plague modern society. Despite effective antibiotics for treatment of the infection, it continues to be a major health problem throughout the world.

Gonorrhea is caused by the bacterium *Neisseria gonorrhoeae*. This organism is highly sensitive to ultraviolet light, drying, heat, and disinfectants and is therefore transmitted primarily by intimate human contact. Genital or oral-genital contact is generally required for disease transmission.

In the male, symptoms of gonorrhea generally develop three to five days after exposure. The male is much more frequently symptomatic than the female and usually seeks medical attention because of urethritis. In this condition, there is painful inflammation of the urethra, the tube coming from the bladder. In addition, bacteria may travel into the male reproductive system, causing inflammation of the epididymis and prostate gland, which are involved in the storage, nourishment, and mobilization of sperm. Scarring, secondary to an infection in this portion of the reproductive tract, may cause sterility.

Twenty percent of women with gonorrhea will not know that they have the infection. Unless they have a prepregnancy evaluation (cervical culture), these patients will not be diagnosed until the first prenatal visit. The remaining 80 percent can manifest gonorrhea in the following ways: 1) vaginal irritation with discharge similar to other vaginal infections; 2) pelvic inflammatory disease (PID), a serious infection of the fallopian tubes that may result in severe scarring and destruction of the tubes and may make conception more difficult or impossible and ectopic pregnancy more likely; and 3) rashes and arthritis.

Once diagnosed, gonorrhea can be effectively treated with antibiotics. Unfortunately, damage to the fallopian tubes cannot be reversed by medication. Traditionally, penicillin was the drug of choice for treatment of gonorrhea. Now, however, because of increasing bacterial resistance to penicillin, other drugs may also be required.

The organism that causes gonorrhea does not usually cross the placenta. It is, however, capable of infecting the baby during passage through the birth canal. Infection in the newborn is most commonly manifested by conjuncti-vitis, an inflammation of one or both eyes. This infection may cause significant eye damage if not treated adequately.

Syphilis

The venereal disease syphilis has frequently been called the great imitator. This illness produces a myriad of problems that frequently simulate other disease processes. Syphilis poses danger not only to infected adults but also to the fetus. Blood screening programs have helped to make this disease very uncommon today.

Syphilis is caused by a spirochete (a spiral-shaped microorganism) known as *Treponema pallidum*. This organism is not found in food, air, water, or insects. Humans are its primary host, and it is capable of living outside the body only for very short periods of time (it is usually killed by drying within one hour). Syphilis is therefore usually transmitted by intimate contact and enters the body through tiny breaks in the skin. Although usually transmitted by sexual intercourse, it may be spread by kissing if an active lesion is present. It is *very rarely* transmitted by eating utensils, cups, or clothing.

There are three stages of syphilitic infection. The primary phase begins one week to two months after contact with an infected person and is manifested by a lesion known as a chancre. This sore, usually single in nature, appears on the external genitalia, the cervix, or on the membranes of the mouth or genital tract. It is smooth at its base and is painless. The chancre lasts one to fourteen days and then heals, with or without treatment.

Approximately two months to two years after the primary phase of syphilis, the second stage begins. Symptoms in the secondary stage include a flu-like illness, swollen lymph nodes, skin rashes, and white patches within the mouth.

A large percentage of individuals with secondary syphilis, if untreated, will enter the tertiary phase of the illness. The organism emerges from the nervous system and may destroy many organs. The skin, bone, intestine, central nervous system, and cardiovascular system are all at risk, and death is a frequent outcome.

Because of the wide range of symptoms seen in syphilis and the intermittent quiet phases of the disease, infection may go undetected. Therefore, all couples must have a blood test in order to get a marriage license, and state laws require a blood test for syphilis of all pregnant women. Obviously, there is an advantage to doing this test even before pregnancy begins.

This screening test, called the VDRL or RPR, is not specific for syphilis; that is, a positive result may occur due to other, noninfectious factors. A patient with a negative VDRL or RPR need not undergo further testing; however, a positive test result indicates that more specific testing should be performed. The FTA (fluorescent treponemal antibody) test is specific for the diagnosis of syphilis. Blood is drawn from the patient and immunological techniques are utilized to confirm or deny the diagnosis of syphilis.

Penicillin is effective therapy for syphilis. This antibiotic will not harm the fetus and may therefore be used in pregnant patients. Treatment of syphilis before the second trimester of pregnancy is highly effective in preventing harmful effects to the fetus. As one might expect, syphilis treated before pregnancy poses no threat to a future pregnancy. If there is an allergy to penicillin, other antibiotics can be prescribed for treatment.

The spirochetes that cause syphilis are capable of crossing the placenta during pregnancy, thus infecting the fetus. A woman with syphilis treated adequately in the first trimester can be relatively confident that the organism has not harmed her fetus. Once a fetus has become infected, a wide range of adverse effects is possible, including miscarriage, premature labor, fetal growth retardation, and stillbirth. Sometimes infants are born in apparently good health and later develop signs of the infection, including abnormal skin, notched teeth, nasal malformations, and deafness.

Herpes Simplex

Herpes simplex virus (HSV) is a sexually transmitted virus. Herpes type I is classically associated with oral lesions (fever blisters), and type II with genital lesions. Although the person infected forms specific antibodies against the virus, it is not eliminated by this immune response. It persists in a latent form and can periodically reactivate. HSV-II is the agent primarily responsible for genital infections. During the primary infection, vesicles (blisters) form. There may also be systemic symptoms such as malaise, myalgia (muscular pain), and fever. The ulcers usually persist for seven to ten days. Episodic recurrence of the active lesions can occur. These lesions are usually fewer and less painful. Virus is shed from the lesion during recurrences and may be shed in asymptomatic people. The primary infection can be treated with a medicine called acyclovir, which decreases the severity of the symptoms and the length of the attack. It may also be used on a continuous basis to prevent recurrences. However, once the medication is stopped, the recurrences may resume.

If a pregnant woman or her partner has a history of a previous genital infection or has a primary infection during pregnancy, she should be screened for active infection. According to the November 1988 bulletin of the American College of Obstetricians and Gynecologists, there is no need to do weekly cultures for herpes. If a recent culture is positive or there is a genital lesion suggestive of herpes present at the onset of labor, the infant should be delivered by cesarean section to prevent passage through the infected birth canal. Infection of a newborn with herpes can be extremely serious. The virus can attack multiple organ systems, including the lungs, liver, and brain. It can result in the death of the infant or in serious long-term impairment.

Human Papillomavirus

The medical literature is replete with evidence that a particular group of viruses, the human papillomaviruses (HPV), are sexually transmitted. Within this viral group, there are many different subtypes, each capable of causing a unique disease, for example, common warts, plantar warts, flat warts, laryngeal papillomas (growths in the vocal cords of infants infected at birth), condyloma acuminata (genital warts), and cervical intraepithelial neoplasia (a precancerous change in the cervix).

This group of viruses is important to those preparing for pregnancy because it commonly infects individuals at the peak age of sexual activity (average age is twenty-four years). The overall incidence of infection in the general population is approximately 3 percent. The virus tends to infect people who engage in sexual activity at a young age and who have multiple sexual partners.

Condyloma acuminata, commonly known as genital warts, is caused by the HPV. The virus, capable of invading genital tissue, including the cervix, vagina, and vulva, induces changes in the normal architecture, causing the formation of a variety of types of warts. These warts are frequently asymptomatic; they may be detected by Pap smear or may be visible to the naked eye. Better visualization of the warts for diagnostic purposes may be accomplished using the colposcope (a low-powered office microscope used to examine living tissue) and biopsy.

Once the diagnosis of condyloma acuminata is made, treatment is initiated in one of several forms. Nonpregnant women may be treated with a chemical known as podophyllin, which is applied directly to the warts. Several treatments may be required. Electrocautery or laser therapy may be used in the pregnant or nonpregnant patient. After the initial treatment, patients are instructed to: 1) maintain hygiene with Betadine soap to the genital area for six months; 2) have their partner use a condom for six months to prevent the spread of condyloma between partners; 3) maintain close follow-up until all warts have disappeared; and 4) have their partner examined and treated as necessary.

Condyloma acuminata should be treated before delivery because the warts may grow enough to cause mechanical obstruction of the birth canal, and because infants born to infected mothers may develop laryngeal papillomas.

AIDS

A particularly devastating disease that can infect pregnant patients is acquired immune deficiency syndrome (AIDS) caused by the HIV virus. Both men and women are susceptible to the virus. The HIV virus attacks a type of lymphocyte (a kind of white blood cell) in the bloodstream. This type of lymphocyte is called a helper T cell. This cell is very important in immune response; therefore, the hallmark of AIDS is a profound and irreversible suppression of the body's immune defense system.

The virus is present in the blood, semen, and saliva of persons who are infected. Infection is caused by intimate contact with an infected person. Although occasional infection of health care workers and family members of AIDS patients has been documented, these cases are very rare. The first cases of AIDS were reported to the Centers for Disease Control in 1981. Since then, infection with the virus has spread rapidly — mainly in large cities among homosexuals, prostitutes, and intravenous drug abusers. In pregnancy, transmission of AIDS to the newborn infant can occur at the time of birth and in utero prior to birth through transplacental infection. The majority of persons in this country who are infected with the AIDS virus have not yet developed the disease. When or if an infected person will develop AIDS is currently unknown, but it is considered that the disease will develop in most infected individuals.

Within the last several years, mass screening of donor blood and plasma for the HIV antibody has been introduced nationwide. Screening of blood products has significantly decreased the risk of developing AIDS from transfusion; however, the risk is still not zero because an individual can be infected several weeks before an antibody is detectable.

Control of the HIV virus will be a difficult task. Research is currently being directed toward drugs to treat patients who already have the disease and to develop a vaccine to protect uninfected persons. It is estimated that development of a vaccine, if successful, will not be accomplished in the foreseeable future. Presently, the best means of control of the AIDS virus is to practice "safe sex," including using condoms. Condoms are believed to significantly decrease the transmission rate of the AIDS virus.

Sexually transmitted diseases pose a threat to pregnancy. Most of the diseases can be detected before pregnancy by relatively simple tests, usually blood tests or swabs from the genital tract, and most sexually transmitted diseases can be effectively treated. However, the treatment is best done before pregnancy to avoid any harm to the fetus from the medication or the disease itself. In some instances, follow-up tests during pregnancy will be necessary.

[13]

Infections in Pregnancy
Kimberly K. Leslie, M.D.

Nine months is a long time. If you add to it the few months when you are planning the pregnancy, you approach one year (the twelve-month pregnancy). It is very unlikely for anyone to go through one year without developing some sort of infection (for example, a viral respiratory infection, urinary tract infection, or vaginitis). Fortunately, these rarely are deleterious to the developing fetus. A few infections, however, can have a harmful effect, so it is very important to understand which ones pose a risk to the fetus as well as the magnitude of that risk.

INFECTIONS occurring in pregnancy may have different implications because two patients, the mother and the fetus, may be affected. A knowledge of a few of the more common infectious agents and the means by which these are treated in pregnancy will help you to understand and react to symptoms in a more timely manner.

Bacterial Infections

The most common sites for bacterial infections in pregnancy are the urinary and genital tracts. The detection, treatment, and implications of three sexually transmitted bacterial infections — chlamydia, gonorrhea, and syphilis — have already been described in the preceding chapter.

URINARY TRACT INFECTIONS

The physiologic changes that occur in the urinary tract place the pregnant woman at risk for acquiring an infection. Many times, the bacterial infection will be asymptomatic, causing no pain. Four to eighteen percent of all pregnant patients will have asymptomatic bacteriuria at any given time. Women who are at high risk for asymptomatic bacteriuria include those of increased age and parity (number of babies delivered), those with sickle cell trait, and those with a previous history of urinary tract infections. Screening is recommended for all pregnant women on their first prenatal visit to rule out asymptomatic bacteriuria. Some authorities recommend that patients be re-screened at various intervals during the pregnancy, depending on their risk factors. If patients with asymptomatic urinary tract infections are not identified and treated, they are at risk for developing pyelonephritis, or infection of the kidneys. Approximately 30 percent of patients with untreated bacteria in the bladder will develop pyelonephritis.

Various bacteria are responsible for these bladder infections; however, the most common are those that are normal flora of the intestinal tract. If the infection is confined to the urinary bladder (a condition called cystitis), it can be adequately treated with oral antibiotics, most of which are safe in pregnancy when prescribed by your physician. If the infection has ascended to affect the kidneys, hospitalization and intravenous antibiotics will be required to eradicate it completely. The signs and symptoms of a urinary tract infection can include fever, flank pain, and symptoms associated with urgency, frequency, and pain with urination.

For patients who have had previous urinary tract infections, we recommend a repeat urine culture on a monthly basis to rule out recurrence. It is important to treat bacterial infections during pregnancy because these can predispose to premature labor and premature delivery.

GROUP B BETA HEMOLYTIC STREPTOCOCCUS

Probably the bacterium most commonly associated with complications in pregnancy is Group B beta hemolytic streptococcus (GBS). GBS is the leading cause of bacterial infection of the blood and meninges (covering of the brain) in the first two months of life. The neonate acquires the infection from the mother during birth or following rupture of the membranes when the mother harbors the bacteria in her genital tract. It is estimated that approximately 50 percent of infants born to mothers who are colonized by these bacteria will themselves become colonized, although only about 1 percent become ill. GBS is a common bacterium, with between 5 and 25 percent of women and men harboring it in their genital tracts. Screening tests can identify these patients. Although numerous attempts have been made in the past to eradicate the bacteria during prenatal care, most of these have been unsuccessful. The majority of the women become recolonized even when their partners are treated as well. At the present time, some authorities recommend screening all patients for colonization with GBS, and treating them when they go into labor to prevent transmission to the fetus. Others recommend that screening is not indicated but that treatment should be given for high-risk situations such as premature rupture of the membranes or prematurity. This bacterium is sensitive to most forms of penicillin, and for those who are allergic to penicillin, other relatively safe antibiotics can be substituted.

Viral Infections

In addition to herpes simplex virus and the AIDS virus, which are discussed in the previous chapter, several other viral infections can be of concern during pregnancy.

CHICKENPOX

Varicella zoster virus (chickenpox) is a common childhood disease that results in a fever, rash, and malaise. The rash starts as macules (small red patches) and progresses to blisters, then pustules, and then scabs. Varicella infections among adults are unusual but when they occur can result in a severe pneumonia.

Maternal varicella infection during the first half of pregnancy can produce congenital anomalies including scarring of the skin, limb abnormalities, and ocular abnormalities. However, the risk of this syndrome is considered to be small. If exposed to varicella, nonimmune pregnant women should be given varicella zoster immune globulin within four days of exposure to protect the mother.

If a pregnant woman develops chickenpox within five days of delivery or up to five days after delivery, the neonate can develop a severe varicella infection. These infants should receive varicella zoster immune globulin.

CYTOMEGALOVIRUS

Cytomegalovirus (CMV) is also a member of the herpes virus group. It is the most common cause of intrauterine infection, and 5 to 10 percent of the infants exposed to this virus in utero will develop neurologic aftereffects. Ninety percent of women with primary or recurrent infection are totally asymptomatic. The remaining 10 percent have a very mild viral-like syndrome.

CMV infections acquired in utero are of concern. Congenital infections can result from either primary or recurrent maternal infection, but they are usually associated with a primary infection. Exposure to secretions of persons excreting the virus can result in maternal infection. Infants who acquired CMV infection during the first trimester are most severely affected. Most infants who acquired the infection during the third trimester are normal.

Infants born with clinically evident disease have a poor prognosis. They have central nervous system and perceptual disabilities, which can result in severe mental retardation. Ninety percent of infants born with the disease are normal at birth but may have subsequent abnormal neurologic development, usually manifested only by high-frequency hearing loss.

Cytomegalovirus is not curable. Several vaccines are under investigation, but none is available for clinical use. There are no set guidelines for the prevention of CMV infection in pregnancy. Routine screening does not give helpful information, since maternal antibodies do not prevent recurrent infections. Unfortunately, it is difficult to avoid being exposed to CMV. The virus is present everywhere but is especially common among children. Prospective parents who work in hospitals and schools should practice careful hand washing. In adults, CMV infection is often asymptomatic; however, a new or acute infection can usually be documented by blood studies.

RUBELLA

Rubella (measles) is a virus that causes a mild illness with fever, arthralgia (joint pain), and rash. Due to development of the rubella vaccine in 1969, the incidence of congenital rubella syndrome in the United States has dropped significantly. The risk of having a child with congenital rubella syndrome as a consequence of maternal infection in the first trimester is over 20 percent. After five months gestation, maternal infection does not appear to have an adverse effect on the fetus. Abnormalities seen in the congenital syndrome include heart defects, cataracts, and deafness. Once immunity has been established, reinfection does not occur. All women considering pregnancy should be tested for immunity and if not immune, they should be vaccinated.

HEPATITIS

Hepatitis viruses cause inflammation of the liver. There are three main types of hepatitis: A, B, and non-A, non-B. Hepatitis A is usually mild and can be prevented by giving the exposed person immune serum globulin. The non-A, non-B virus can be contracted through a blood transfusion and causes liver damage similar to that of A and B hepatitis, and is also a generally mild disease. The major problem is hepatitis B, because of the fact that certain individuals are chronic carriers of the virus and transmission to the fetus can occur. The Centers for Disease Control recommend that all mothers be screened for hepatitis B during pregnancy.

If the mother has an acute infection and the infant develops the disease, it is usually mild; however, many of these children become chronic carriers of the virus. If the mother is a chronic carrier and the infant develops the disease, it can be quite severe or even fatal. These infants also commonly become carriers and often develop cirrhosis or cancer of the liver later in life. Prevention of the carrier states in the infant can be accomplished in many cases by giving the infant hepatitis B immune globulin and the hepatitis B vaccine. Adults at risk for contracting hepatitis B should also be immunized.

Persons who are at risk for hepatitis B and non-A, non-B include intravenous drug users who share needles, homosexuals, and persons with multiple sex partners. For these types of hepatitis, it is generally believed that the virus must reach the bloodstream to be infective (serum transmission). Hepatitis A can be transmitted through contact with infected body secretions, and serum, or blood, contact is not necessary.

Therefore, hepatitis A can be transmitted to anyone who comes into relatively casual contact with an infected person.

Protozoal Infections

Toxoplasmosis is an illness caused by a protozoan, *Toxoplasma gondii*. This organism is found in many animals, but the only definitive host is the cat. Humans can acquire the infection by eating the raw or undercooked meat of infected animals, especially lamb, or by contact with the feces of infected cats. The infection in the adult is usually mild and is a flu-like illness. Fever, sore throat, and a rash may appear, but the infection may also be asymptomatic. If an infection occurs during pregnancy, 30 to 60 percent of the fetuses will become infected. In the majority of the newborns, the infection is subclinical (without detectable effect). A small minority will have evidence of serious disease, including calcifications in the brain, convulsions, jaundice, and ocular problems. This can lead to mental retardation and blindness. If the infection occurs during the first trimester, the likelihood of transmission to the fetus is low but the effects are greater. The possibility of transmission to the fetus during the third trimester is higher, but the infections are almost always subclinical.

If a pregnant woman acquires toxoplasmosis, she can be treated with medications. There is evidence that treatment reduces the frequency of fetal infection. However, prevention of infection is the best way to avoid problems: do not eat undercooked meats, wash your hands after handling a cat, and have someone else change the litter box.

The most important thing for prospective parents to remember is that despite the horror stories, infections that result in significant fetal damage are very rare. The vast majority of viral illnesses will not result in complications, and bacterial infections are treatable and curable.

[14]

High-Risk Pregnancy
Kimberly K. Leslie, M.D.

Most pregnancies end successfully with a healthy baby. However, approximately 10 percent to 15 percent of established pregnancies have a maternal or fetal factor that threatens the favorable outcome. These are termed high-risk pregnancies. Some of their contributing factors can be identified before pregnancy. For example, if the mother has a condition such as chronic hypertension or insulin-dependent diabetes mellitus, she is at risk. Other high-risk situations develop during the course of pregnancy, such as premature separation of the placenta or premature rupture of the fetal membranes. By understanding these high-risk factors, you will be better able to minimize their effect or to cope if problems arise.

FOR THE VAST MAJORITY of women, pregnancy is uncomplicated, and labor and delivery culminate in the birth of a healthy newborn. Only a relatively small percentage of couples will have to cope with problems associated with the process. This chapter will discuss some of the complications that place a pregnancy in the high-risk category, but the infrequency of these events should be kept in mind. For purposes of presentation, the risk factors can be divided into those presented by maternal disease (usually preexisting) and those arising from pregnancy-related complications.

Risk Resulting from Maternal Disease

A pregnancy is considered high risk if the mother has a major medical illness, though even in the presence of maternal disease, with proper management, the pregnancy outcome is likely to be good. What follows is a discussion of several of the more common disorders and their effect upon pregnancy. This is only a partial list of the many medical conditions that can have an impact. Patients with known disorders should seek directed preconception counseling about the effect of the disease upon pregnancy and, conversely, the effect of pregnancy upon the disease and its possible progression. Entering the pregnancy in the best condition possible will have many benefits as the gestation proceeds.

DIABETES

Diabetes is a common complication of pregnancy, as hormonal changes unmask latent tendencies toward this endocrinologic dysfunction. Diabetes is a condition caused by inadequate secretion of the hormone insulin from the pancreas. The function of insulin is to decrease the blood sugar (glucose) to a normal level after carbohydrate consumption and to allow glucose to enter the cells of the body so that it can be utilized. In the absence of adequate pancreatic secretion of insulin, blood sugar rises to harmful levels. Several of the hormones secreted by the placenta counteract the effects of insulin, making it necessary for the mother's pancreas to secrete at least 30 percent more insulin to maintain adequate glucose control during pregnancy. Therefore, women who are known diabetics prior to pregnancy and those who become so during pregnancy (gestational diabetics) need careful monitoring. Diabetes can be associated with the birth of larger-than-average infants who need special monitoring in the nursery. Maternal diabetes predisposes the fetus to a higher-than-average chance of stillbirth late in gestation and to an increased risk for malformations occurring early in gestation. These risks can be significantly decreased by careful prepregnancy and prenatal glucose control, which entails selective dieting supplemented by additional insulin as necessary. The other endocrinologic disorders, such as thyroid and parathyroid diseases, are usually associated with good pregnancy outcomes when well controlled.

HEART DISEASE

It is estimated that 1 percent of all pregnancies are complicated by maternal heart disease. Since the outcome depends largely upon the type of cardiac disease present, it is important that the correct diagnosis be made prior to pregnancy. The most common form of heart disease in the United States results from rheumatic fever, which usually affects the mitral valve.

In the absence of severe and debilitating disease, the outcome in most pregnancies is good. It is recommended that patients with valvular heart disease receive antibiotics before and after delivery to prevent further damage to the heart valves from bacteria that could enter the maternal circulation during delivery. This antibiotic regimen is also recommended by some experts for patients with mitral valve prolapse. Mitral valve prolapse is the most common congenital heart defect affecting young women and is associated with a specific murmur suggestive of a floppy mitral valve. The pregnancy outcome in mitral valve prolapse is usually good. Women who have other diseases linked to severe valvular damage may be advised to have surgical correction or replacement of the valve prior to attempting pregnancy. There are at least two types of heart disease in which the maternal mortality rate is so high that pregnancy is not recommended: Eisenmenger syndrome and primary pulmonary hypertension. In any event, a complete cardiac evaluation prior to pregnancy is necessary for women with cardiac disease of any kind. The inheritance pattern of congenital heart disease is most often multifactorial (due to a combination of genetic and environmental influences), but there is a 2 to 4 percent risk to the fetus of inheriting the defect if its mother has congenital heart disease. Therefore, these fetuses should be carefully evaluated in utero for the presence of structural heart abnormalities. Major malformations can usually be detected by sonography at sixteen to eighteen weeks gestation.

Hypertension

Mothers with chronic hypertension, or high blood pressure, are considered high risk and require special care during pregnancy. The blood pressure should be controlled with antihypertensives when necessary. Chronic hypertension is associated with vascular changes that can lead to placental insufficiency, causing problems like intrauterine growth retardation. Therefore, periodic testing to assess health as pregnancy progresses is the mainstay of management.

Epilepsy

The most common neurologic disorder seen in our patients at Georgetown is epilepsy. These patients usually enter pregnancy with a known history of recurrent seizures. Most physicians feel strongly that medication should be continued throughout gestation to prevent the occurrence of seizures, which can put both mother and fetus at risk. It is important for anyone with this disorder to be placed on adequate doses of the safest drugs possible prior to becoming pregnant. Although two anticonvulsants should be avoided in pregnancy (valproic acid and trimethadione), the most commonly used drugs have an acceptable risk-benefit ratio. Medication levels should be monitored and adjusted as necessary to maintain a therapeutic range. Most anticonvulsants are folic acid antagonists, and dietary supplementation of this important vitamin is particularly important for the pregnant patient with epilepsy.

COLLAGEN VASCULAR DISORDERS

The collagen vascular, or rheumatic, diseases are a group of disorders that affect multiple organ systems. The most commonly seen disorders from this group include rheumatoid arthritis, which affects about 2 percent of the population, and systemic lupus erythematosus (SLE), which affects about 1 in 1,000. These disorders are autoimmune in nature, meaning that the body is mounting an immune response against itself. Pregnancy does not appear to have an adverse effect on the majority of patients with collagen vascular disease; however, some do experience worsening symptoms. Exacerbations may occasionally occur in the immediate postpartum period. In SLE, certain antibodies, called lupus anticoagulants, may be associated with an increased rate of spontaneous abortion. Fifteen percent of patients with SLE do develop these antibodies, and successful treatment of patients in this group who have experienced recurrent miscarriages has been reported. The incidence of premature birth and stillbirth is increased in patients with SLE, and antepartum testing to assess fetal health is advisable. The neonate of the mother with SLE is also at some increased risk for developing heart block, a disorder of the cardiac conduction system. When the diagnosis of heart block is made early, successful neonatal therapy is often possible.

Risk Resulting from Pregnancy-Related Complications

Mothers who are healthy entering pregnancy may experience one or more complications that place them in the high-risk category. Some of the most commonly occurring complications include premature labor, premature rupture of the fetal membranes, and pre-eclampsia.

PREMATURE LABOR

Premature onset of uterine contractions can lead to labor and the delivery of a premature infant. In the majority of cases, the reason for the early onset of labor is unknown. Due to advancements in neonatal intensive care technology, the premature infant born today has a much better chance of surviving and leading a normal life than would have been possible in decades past. However, we have been unable to significantly reduce the percentage of infants born prematurely. The complete mechanism for the onset of labor is unknown at present. Therefore, medical intervention techniques are all too often unsuccessful.

It is normal for the pregnant woman to have occasional episodes of uterine activity. These are called Braxton-Hicks contractions, and they may be painful, but they do not lead to cervical dilatation, which is the hallmark of true labor. They are more common in the third trimester of pregnancy but can occur earlier. The challenge for the patient and the obstetrician is to determine in a timely manner whether the contractions experienced will lead to progressive cervical shortening (effacement) and dilatation, that is, to true labor. We recommend to our patients that any significant increase in uterine activity be reported. In patients who are remote from term (earlier than thirty-seven weeks), regular contractions that occur over a span of several hours and could be a warning sign of impending premature labor. A trip to the hospital's labor and delivery unit for monitoring will usually settle the issue, and therapy can be instituted if necessary. Treatment is more likely to be successful if initiated early.

PREMATURE RUPTURE OF THE MEMBRANES

Premature labor is commonly associated with premature rupture of the fetal membranes (the amnion and chorion), which releases amniotic fluid. Again, the cause of this disorder is usually obscure. We believe that premature rupture may be associated with the presence of certain types of bacteria in the cervix which can attach to and weaken the membranes. However, just as with premature labor, the initiating event may be unknown. In the absence of any signs of infection, cautious observation is recommended if early rupture occurs. Patients are usually hospitalized and monitored for signs of maternal or fetal complications. If there is infection or fetal distress, delivery is indicated. In most instances, vaginal delivery can be accomplished; with situations like breech (rear end first) presentation or unripe cervix, a cesarean section may be necessary.

PRE-ECLAMPSIA

Pre-eclampsia is a condition that includes increased blood pressure, protein in the urine, and significant tissue swelling (edema). Pre-eclampsia is also associated with increased neural irritability, manifesting itself as reflex excitability, which can lead to seizures. If seizures occur, the disease is considered to have progressed to eclampsia. The cause of pre-eclampsia is unknown. There is no cure for the disease short of delivery, but in many cases, its progression can be controlled to allow for the continuation of the pregnancy for days or weeks. For the most part, pre-eclampsia is a disease of first pregnancies. It can cause prematurity, intrauterine growth retardation, and, in the worst cases, even fetal death. It may increase the chance of preeclampsia in subsequent gestations.

As can be seen from a quick review of pregnancy-related complications, much work needs to be done to better define the causes of these disorders. However, improved antepartum and neonatal management has resulted in a steadily falling maternal and neonatal complication rate. It can now be safely stated that the majority of established pregnancies, even when complicated, result in the birth of a baby mature enough to survive.

[15]

Ultrasonography
Kimberly K. Leslie, M.D., and
John J. Schruefer, M.D.

Before the development of X rays, the practice of internal medicine was less exact. To determine the presence or absence of a problem in the lungs, for instance, the physician listened to the chest with a stethoscope and percussed the chest wall. With the advent of X rays, the accuracy of diagnosis immediately increased. However, even though X rays enabled physicians to make more accurate diagnoses, they still did not throw away their stethoscopes.

A similar situation has occurred in obstetrics. Prior to the advent of diagnostic ultrasound, the size of the uterus was determined by a pelvic examination in the first trimester of pregnancy and subsequently was determined by the height of the uterus as it grew. Now, with the use of diagnostic ultrasonography, the early diagnosis of pregnancy can be made visually, and the presence of the beating fetal heart can be identified. Subsequently, the anatomical aspects of the fetus can be determined, indicating normal or abnormal development, and much other important information can be ascertained. Today, ultrasonography is an important diagnostic tool in evaluating any pregnancy. The obstetrician is capable of establishing the correct gestational age, diagnosing the presence of twins, and indicating when there are certain congenital malformations or abnormal fetal growth patterns. There are, of course, many other applications for diagnostic ultrasound that have added precision to the evaluation of pregnancy.

Ultrasonography is also an extremely important tool for evaluation of the pelvic organs prior to the onset of pregnancy, and it is commonly used in gynecologic evaluation today. By this we do not mean that ultrasonography is used in all gynecologic examinations, but it does have many specific applications. Thus, ultrasonography can be extremely helpful in making gynecologic assessments and, in many instances, in avoiding surgical procedures as a means of diagnosis.

D IAGNOSTIC ULTRASONOGRAPHY has revolutionized the field of obstetrics. This new technology, which grew out of the use of sonar in World War II, was put to medical use in the 1940s. Sonography has since been found to be an excellent tool for imaging a fetus within the pregnant uterus. Because ultrasound is such a valuable tool for assessing the pelvic anatomy and following fetal development, many women will have a study performed during their pregnancy. This chapter will review the mechanical principles of sonography and discuss its many clinical uses — all of which will be helpful to understand when preparing for pregnancy.

The Mechanics of Ultrasonography

High-frequency sound waves are used to produce sonographic images. The frequency of these waves is so high that they cannot be heard by the human ear, hence the name ultrasound. An electrical current is passed through the sound emitter, called a transducer. The transducer is made of a special material, such as crystal or ceramic, which is capable of producing sound waves from electrical energy. It converts that energy to molecular motion which, in turn, produces very high frequency sound waves. The sound waves thus produced pass through the body and are reflected back to the transducer. They are then reconverted to electrical energy, which is amplified and processed to create a visual image.

An ultrasound scan is done with the patient lying flat on an examination table. Preferably, her bladder should be full for a gynecologic scan or an exam early in pregnancy (this reflects the sound waves better). A liquid gel is placed on the abdomen to serve as a conducting medium, then the transducer is passed over the abdomen. The sound waves bounce off structures in the abdomen and pelvis, are received by the transducer, and are then converted to a black and white image on a television screen.

Alternatively, to image structures deep in the pelvis, a vaginal transducer may be used. In this way, the sound waves do not have to pass through the abdominal wall. This technique is especially useful to determine when the ovarian follicle is ready to ovulate, to detect an ectopic (tubal) pregnancy, and for early observation of the normal pregnancy.

The ultrasound transducer actually produces sound just 0.1 percent of the time. During the remaining 99.9 percent of the time, the transducer is only listening for reflected sound waves. This fact is important to consider when judging the potentially harmful effects of a sonographic study on the developing fetus. The study is less likely to produce damage if the energy is emitted for short periods of time.

The Use of Ultrasound in Gynecology

The clinical use of ultrasound is not limited to pregnancy. Ultrasound can be used to observe the normal internal female anatomy as well as to diagnose abnormalities of the female genital tract. In a normal gynecological sonogram, the uterus as well as the ovaries can usually be visualized. The normal follicle (cyst) within an ovary that contains the developing egg can be visualized by ultrasound. Thus, sonography is a useful tool for the evaluation of women taking fertility drugs to induce ovulation.

Some other types of cysts on the ovary are easily identifiable by sonography. Many cysts or masses have characteristic images, and careful ultrasound evaluation can obviate the need for surgery. Ultrasound has also been helpful in evaluating patients who have chronic pelvic pain or possible pelvic inflammatory disease. Abnormalities of the uterus such as uterine fibroids and septae can be seen by ultrasound. Fibroids, which are muscular tumors that grow on the uterus, are usually benign and are quite common in the general population. The diagnosis of a septate uterus (when the uterus is divided by a partition) can be important in the workup of patients who have experienced recurrent and unexplained pregnancy losses.

The Use of Ultrasound in Obstetrics

Sonography in the first trimester of pregnancy can be used to diagnose, confirm, and date a pregnancy.

The presence of an intrauterine gestation can be visualized four weeks after conception, or six weeks after the last normal menstrual period began. This first ultrasonographic image of the pregnancy consists of a simple sac seen within the uterus. By five weeks postconception, the outline of the embryo should be seen. The embryo can be measured and an approximate gestational age can be determined. By six weeks postconception, the fetal heart can be seen beating within the chest of the embryo. This fact is very helpful in distinguishing pregnancies that are developing normally at this point from those that are destined to abort.

Bleeding in the first trimester of the pregnancy can be

evaluated by sonography. The presence of a living conceptus in the uterus makes the possibility of spontaneous abortion, or "miscarriage," less likely. It also rules out the possibility that the bleeding was caused by a very dangerous type of pregnancy: an ectopic pregnancy. In an ectopic pregnancy, the fetus has implanted somewhere outside the uterine cavity, usually in a fallopian tube. The danger lies in the fact that the fallopian tube cannot expand to accommodate the growing embryo, and thus may be de-

Figure 15-1. Typical Sonograms

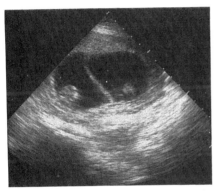

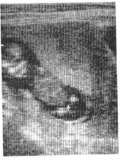

A. Gestational sacs showing twin fetuses at ten weeks gestation.

B. Sonogram of fetus demonstrates the technique of measuring the crown-rump length of 66 millimeters, which corresponds to thirteen weeks gestation.

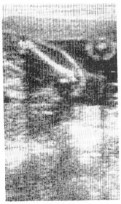

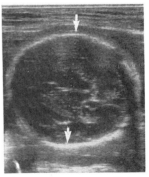

C. Fetal femur (thigh) bone measurement of 45 millimeters corresponds to twenty-three weeks gestation.

D. Sonogram of fetal head showing technique for measuring the width of the head (biparietal diameter), which measures 66 millimeters and corresponds to twenty-six weeks gestation.

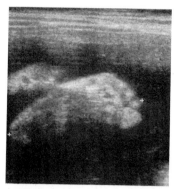

E. Sonogram showing the right fetal foot, which measures 71 millimeters.

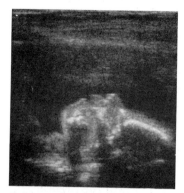

F. Sonogram showing fetal head in profile.

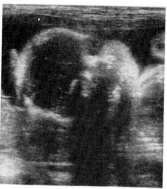

G. Sonogram showing fetal face.

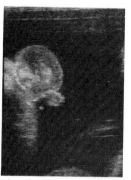

H. The scrotum and penis are visualized on this male fetus.

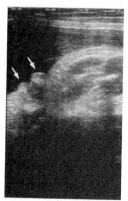

I. Labia majora (arrows) are visualized, indicating a female fetus.

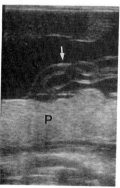

J. Sonogram of a posteriorly implanted placenta (P) showing the umbilical cord insertion (arrow).

stroyed by the pregnancy growing within. If undetected, an ectopic pregnancy often leads to severe bleeding and is a major cause of maternal mortality in this country. Ultrasonography is helpful in making the diagnosis so that steps may be taken to terminate the pregnancy, thus reducing damage to the mother's reproductive system and ending the risk of hemorrhage.

There are many other indications for diagnostic ultrasonography during pregnancy. If the uterus appears too large for the expected dates, a sonogram will be ordered to see if twins are present and to confirm the true gestational age of the pregnancy. Conversely, if the uterus is too small, sonography can be used to confirm the due date of the pregnancy and assess fetal growth.

From fifteen to twenty-five weeks gestation, the measurement of the fetal head width (biparietal diameter) and the fetal femur length are accurate ways to determine gestational age. If a mother is uncertain of the date of her last normal menstrual period or if she is going to have a repeat cesarean section before the onset of labor, sonography is very useful to determine correct gestational age at this early point in the pregnancy. Later in pregnancy, measurements to determine gestational age are less accurate due to the wide biological variation in fetal size.

The ability to diagnose many congenital malformations is another advantage of the use of sonography during pregnancy. The recommended time for performing a screening sonogram is between eighteen and twenty weeks of gestation. Prior to this time, some defects will not be detectable. It should be remembered that certain abnormalities will not be diagnosable by ultrasound, even using the best techniques available. These defects include chromosome problems, such as Down syndrome, and subtle structural defects.

Later on, in the second half of the pregnancy, ultrasound

is performed for other indications. One of these is to verify the presentation of the fetus; that is, to ascertain if the fetus is positioned in the uterus with the head down, directed toward the birth canal. Abnormal presentations, such as breech (feet or buttocks first) or transverse lie (sideways), will make the delivery more complicated.

The use of ultrasound to diagnose the cause of bleeding in the first trimester has already been discussed, but it should be remembered that bleeding during any time in pregnancy can be an abnormal event and may require an ultrasound examination. Bleeding during the later months of pregnancy may be due to an abnormal placental location within the uterus. Bleeding may result if the placenta is implanted very low in the uterus overlying part or all of the cervix. This is called a placenta previa and is a potentially serious condition. Another reason for bleeding in the second and third trimester is a placental abruption. In this case, premature separation of the placenta from the uterine wall has occurred. Occasionally, although not commonly, a placental abruption can also be seen by sonography.

Safety and Ultrasound

Since ultrasound has been in use in medicine, numerous studies have been done to investigate the possible detrimental effects caused by passing sound waves through tissue. The theoretical sources of tissue damage may occur as a result of heat production and cavitation by ultrasound energy. Cavitation refers to the generation of tiny gas bubbles within the water component of tissues, which leads to cellular damage. The conclusion of the National Institutes of Health Consensus Development Conference on Obstetrical Ultrasound, after careful consideration of all available scientific studies, was that there was *no* evidence of ultrasound damage to human fetuses at the power levels currently being used in the United States for ultrasound imaging. Follow-up studies of infants exposed in utero to diagnostic ultrasound have not detected any adverse effects. Despite this apparent safety, it remains prudent to state that until further follow-up long-term testing is done, the absolute safety of ultrasound cannot be proven. It is clear, however, that in certain clinical situations, the danger of *not* having an ultrasound may be much greater than the risk of the test.

Seeing the fetus for the first time during an ultrasound examination is a momentous event with positive impact upon both parents. Although a normal study does not guarantee a perfect pregnancy, it can go a long way toward reassuring the parents that things are progressing well. Also, it is clearly documented that visualizing the fetus during sonography promotes parental bonding.

Epilogue

THE PRECEDING CHAPTERS have presented a concept we believe will offer you your best opportunity of improving your chance to have a healthy baby. It makes sense to be in your best physical condition prior to starting pregnancy. In addition, knowing potential beneficial measures like nutrition and exercise as well as what to avoid in the way of foods or medications seems logical.

A couple has innumerable choices to make in the course of having a baby. Considering and discussing these options should provide fun and a sense of constructive sharing as you proceed.

The major factors that should be stressed prior to becoming pregnant are:

education
physical examination
Pap smear
blood evaluation
risk evaluation
genetic considerations
prenatal vitamin supplement with iron

good nutrition
regular exercise
choice of hospital
choice of doctor
financial considerations
good communication with your health care providers

You are embarking on one of life's most fulfilling adventures. Prepare, and make the most of it.

John T. Queenan, M.D.

Readings and Resources

READINGS

General

Brazelton, T. Berry, *On Becoming a Family: The Growth of Attachment.* New York: Delacorte, 1981.

——, *Working and Caring.* Reading, Massachusetts: Addison-Wesley, 1987.

Chamberlain, G., and Lemley, J., *Prepregnancy Care.* Chichester, England: J. Wiley and Sons, 1986.

U.S. Department of Health and Human Services, *Prenatal Care.* DHHS Pub. No. (HRSA) 83–5070. Washington, D.C., 1983.

Queenan, John T., and Queenan, Carrie N., *A New Life.* Boston: Little, Brown, 1986.

Verrilli, G. E., and Mueser, A. M., *While Waiting.* New York: St. Martin's, 1985.

Pregnancy Loss and Grief

Borg, Susan, and Lasker, Judith, *When Pregnancy Fails: Families Coping with Miscarriage, Stillbirth and Infant Death.* Boston: Beacon Press, 1981.

Defrain, J., et al., *Stillbirth — The Invisible Death.* Lexington, Massachusetts: Lexington Books, 1986.

Ilse, Sherokee, *Empty Arms: A Guide to Help Parents and Loved Ones Cope with Miscarriage, Stillbirth and Newborn Death.* Long Lake, Minnesota: Wintergreen Press, 1982.

Ilse, Sherokee, and Burns, Linda Hammer, *Miscarriage: A Shattered Dream*. Long Lake, Minnesota: Wintergreen Press, 1985.

Peppers, L. G., and Knapp, R. J., *How to Go On Living After the Death of a Baby*. Atlanta: Peachtree, 1985.

Schiff, Harriett, *Bereaved Parents*. New York: Crown, 1977.

Schwiebert, P., and Kirk, P., *When Hello Means Good-bye: A Guide for Parents Whose Baby Dies Shortly Before or After Birth*. Portland, Oregon: Perinatal Loss, 1988. (Spanish and English available.)

Children, For and About

Erling, J., and Erling, S., *Our Baby Died. Why?* Wayzata, Minnesota: Pregnancy and Infant Loss Center, 1986.

Grollman, Earl A., *Explaining Death to Children*. Boston: Beacon Press, 1967.

———, *Talking About Death: A Dialogue Between Parents and Child*. Boston: Beacon Press, 1976.

Ilse, Sherokee, and Burns, Linda Hammer, *Sibling Grief . . . After Miscarriage, Stillbirth, or Infant Death*. Wayzata, Minnesota: Pregnancy and Infant Loss Center, 1984.

Lamb, J., and Dodge, N., *Thumpy's Story. Sharing with Thumpy Workbook. Thumpy's Story Coloring Book*. Springfield, Illinois: Prairie Lark Press, 1984–85.

Schaefer, D., and Lyon, C., *How Do We Tell the Children?* Brooklyn: Daniel J. Schaefer Consulting Company, 1985.

Self-Help

Colgrove, Melba, et al., *How to Survive the Loss of a Loved One*. New York: Bantam, 1977.

Grollman, Earl A., *What Helped Me When My Loved One Died*. Boston: Beacon Press, 1981.

———, *Living When a Loved One Has Died*. Boston: Beacon Press, 1981.

Manning, Doug, *Don't Take My Grief Away From Me*, Springfield, Illinois: Creative Marketing, 1984.

Stearns, Ann Kaiser, *Living Through Personal Crisis*. New York: Ballantine Books, 1984.

Westberg, Granger, *Good Grief*. Philadelphia: Fortress Press, 1962.

Subsequent Pregnancy

Halcs, Dianne, and Creasy, Robert K., *New Hope for Problem Pregnancies: Helping Babies Before They're Born.* New York: Harper and Row, 1982.

Ilse, S., and Erling, S., *What Next? After Miscarriage, Stillborn or Infant Death.* Long Lake, Minnesota: Wintergreen Press, 1984.

Schwiebert, P., and Kirk, P., *Still to Be Born.* Portland, Oregon: Perinatal Loss, 1986.

Breast-feeding

Dana, Nancy, and Price, Anne, *The Working Woman's Guide to Breastfeeding.* Deephaven, Minnesota: Meadowbrook, 1987.

Eiger, Marvin S., and Olds, Sally Wendkos, *The Complete Book of Breastfeeding.* New York: Workman Publishing, 1987.

Kamen, Betty, and Kamen, Si, *Total Nutrition for Breast-feeding Mothers.* Boston: Little, Brown, 1986.

Kintzinger, Sheila, *The Experience of Breastfeeding.* Harmondsworth, England: Penguin Books, 1987.

Renkauf, Diane M., and Trause, Mary Anne, *Commonsense Breastfeeding.* New York: Atheneum, 1988.

Pain Management

Jones, Carl, *Mind Over Labor.* New York: Viking Penguin, 1987.

Nutrition and Exercise

Brody, Jane, *Jane Brody's Nutrition Book.* New York: Norton, 1981.

Brown, Judith E., *Nutrition for Your Pregnancy: The University of Minnesota Guide.* New York: New American Library, 1983.

Darden, Ellington, *The Nautilus Woman.* New York: Simon and Schuster, 1983.

Hess, Mary Abbott, and Hunt, Anne Elise, *Pickles and Cream: The Complete Guide to Nutrition During Pregnancy.* New York: McGraw-Hill, 1982.

Shangold, Mona, and Mirkin, Gabe, *The Complete Sports Medicine Book for Women.* New York: Simon and Schuster, 1985.

Winick, Dr. Myron, *Nutrition in Pregnancy.* White Plains, New York: March of Dimes Birth Defects Foundation, 1986.

Medications and Environment

American College of Obstetricians and Gynecologists, *Guidelines for Diagnostic X-ray Examination of Fertile Women.* Chicago: American College of Obstetricians and Gynecologists, 1977.

————, *Guidelines on Pregnancy and Work.* Chicago: American College of Obstetricians and Gynecologists, 1977.

Briggs, G. G., et al., *Drugs in Pregnancy and Lactation: A Reference Guide to Fetal and Neonatal Risk.* Baltimore/London: Williams and Wilkins, 1983.

Heinonen, O. P., et al., *Birth Defects and Drugs in Pregnancy.* Littleton, Massachusetts: Publishing Sciences Group, 1977.

National Council on Radiation Protection and Measurements, *Review of NRCP Radiation Dose Limit for Embryo and Fetus in Occupationally Exposed Women.* Report no. 53. Washington, D.C.: NCRPM, 1977.

Genetics

Goodman, Richard M., *Planning for a Healthy Baby: A Guide to Genetic and Environmental Risks.* New York: Oxford University Press, 1986.

Puck, Sterling M., and Fleming, Jamie P., *Genetics, Environment, and Your Baby.* Santa Fe: Vivigen, 1986.

High-Risk Pregnancies

Queenan, John T., ed., *Management of High-Risk Pregnancies.* Oradell, New Jersey: Medical Economics, 1987.

RESOURCES/INFORMATION CENTERS

American Academy of Pediatrics
P.O. Box 1034
Evanston, Illinois 60204

American Foundation for Maternal and Child Health
30 Beekman Place
New York, New York 10022

American Society for Psychoprophylaxis in Obstetrics (ASPO)
1840 Wilson Boulevard, Suite 204
Arlington, Virginia 22201

American College of Nurse Midwives
1522 K Street, N.W., Suite 1120
Washington, D.C. 20005

American College of Obstetricians and Gynecologists
600 Maryland Avenue, S.W.
Washington, D.C. 20024
(Offers a useful publication, *Planning for Your Pregnancy*.)

Environmental Mutagen, Carcinogen, and Teratogen Information Department
Oak Ridge National Laboratory
Oak Ridge, Tennessee 37830

Environmental Teratology Information Center
P.O. Box 12233
National Institute of Environmental Health Sciences, Mail Drop 18–01
Research Triangle Park, North Carolina 27709

International Childbirth Education Association (ICEA)
Box 20048
Minneapolis, Minnesota 55420

La Leche League International, Inc.
9616 Minneapolis Avenue
Franklin Park, Illinois 60131

March of Dimes Birth Defects Foundation
1275 Mamaroneck Avenue
White Plains, New York 10605

Maternity Center Association, Inc.
48 East 92nd Street
New York, New York 10028

National Center for Education in Maternal and Child Health
38th and R Streets, N.W.
Washington, D.C. 20037
(This center has information about support groups for specific diseases.)

National Women's Health Report
P.O. Box 25307, Georgetown Station
Washington, D.C. 20007
(A newsletter on women's health care.)

Index